Statistics and Quantitative Methods in Nursing

Issues and Strategies for Research and Education

IVO L. ABRAHAM, Ph.D., R.N.
University of Virginia

DEBORAH M. NADZAM, Ph.D., R.N.
Northwestern Memorial Hospital
and Northwestern University

JOYCE J. FITZPATRICK, Ph.D., F.A.A.N.
Case Western Reserve University

1989
W.B. SAUNDERS COMPANY
Harcourt Brace Jovanovich, Inc.
Philadelphia ■ London ■ Toronto ■ Montreal ■ Sydney ■ Tokyo

W.B. SAUNDERS COMPANY
Harcourt Brace Jovanovich, Inc.

The Curtis Center
Independence Square West
Philadelphia, PA 19106-3399

Library of Congress Cataloging-in-Publication Data

Abraham, Ivo Luc.
Statistics and quantitative methods in nursing: issues and strategies for research and education / Ivo L. Abraham, Deborah M. Nadzam, Joyce L. Fitzpatrick.
p. cm.
Includes indexes.
1. Nursing—Research—Statistical methods. I. Nadzam, Deborah M.
II. Fitzpatrick, Joyce L. III. Title.
RT81.5.A26 1989
610.73′015195—dc19
ISBN 0-7216-2224-0

89-30638
CIP

Editor: Thomas Eoyang
Designer: Ellen M. Bodner
Production Manager: Peter Faber
Manuscript Editor: Ronald Harris
Indexer: Ella Shapiro

Statistics and Quantitative Methods in Nursing:
Issues and Strategies for Research and Education   ISBN   0–7216-2224-0

Printed in the United States of America.

Last digit is the print number: 9   8   7   6   5   4   3   2   1

To:
Matthew Abraham
Carrie, Bonnie, and Chrissie Nadzam

CONTRIBUTORS

IVO L. ABRAHAM, Ph.D., R.N.
Department of Behavioral Medicine and Psychiatry
School of Medicine
University of Virginia
Charlottesville, Virginia

JOEL W. AGER, Ph.D.
Professor
Department of Psychology
Wayne State University
Detroit, Michigan

DOROTHY E. BOOTH, Ph.D., R.N.
Assistant Professor
School of Nursing
The University of Michigan
Ann Arbor, Michigan

DONNA R. BROGAN, Ph.D.
Professor
Department of Epidemiology/Biostatistics
Emory University
Atlanta, Georgia

KATHLEEN COEN BUCKWALTER, Ph.D., R.N.
Associate Professor
College of Nursing
University of Iowa
Iowa City, Iowa

CLAUDIA J. COULTON, Ph.D.
Professor
School of Applied Social Science
Case Western Reserve University
Cleveland, Ohio

W. RICHARD COWLING III, Ph.D., R.N.
Associate Professor
Chair, Nursing Science Department
College of Nursing
University of South Carolina
Columbia, South Carolina

KAREN E. DENNIS, Ph.D., R.N.
Instructor and Nursing Research Director
Johns Hopkins University and Francis Scott Key Medical Center
Baltimore, Maryland

SANDRA FERKETICH, Ph.D., R.N.
Associate Professor
Director, Family and Community Health Nursing
College of Nursing
University of Arizona
Tucson, Arizona

JOYCE J. FITZPATRICK, Ph.D., F.A.A.N.
Professor and Dean
Frances Payne Bolton School of Nursing
Case Western Reserve University
Cleveland, Ohio

BEVERLY C. FLYNN, Ph.D., F.A.A.N.
Professor and Chairperson, Department of Community Health Nursing
School of Nursing
Indiana University
Indianapolis, Indiana

MARQUIS D. FOREMAN, Ph.D., R.N.
Postdoctoral Fellow
College of Nursing
University of Illinois at Chicago
Director of Research, Department of Nursing
University of Chicago Hospitals
Chicago, Illinois

JEAN GOEPPINGER, Ph.D., R.N.
Professor and Chair, Community Health Nursing
School of Nursing
University of Michigan
Ann Arbor, Michigan

MARGARET R. GRIER, Ph.D., F.A.A.N.
Professor and Associate Dean for Graduate Studies and Research
College of Nursing
University of Kentucky
Lexington, Kentucky

EDWARD J. HALLORAN, Ph.D., F.A.A.N.
Associate Professor
Frances Payne Bolton School of Nursing
Case Western Reserve University
Cleveland, Ohio

MARY S. HARPER, Ph.D., F.A.A.N.
Coordinator for Long Term Care
National Institute of Mental Health
Rockville, Maryland

LEE-HWA JANE, M.S.N., R.N.
Statistical Consultant
A. R. Jennings Computing Center
Case Western Reserve University
Cleveland, Ohio

MARY M. JIROVEC, Ph.D., R.N.
Assistant Professor
College of Nursing
Wayne State University
Detroit, Michigan

PAUL K. JONES, Ph.D.
Associate Professor
Department of Epidemiology and Biostatistics
Case Western Reserve University
Cleveland, Ohio

SUSAN L. JONES, Ph.D., F.A.A.N.
Professor
School of Nursing
Kent State University
Kent, Ohio

MARYLOU L. KILEY, Ph.D., R.N.
Senior Analyst, Operations Research
Department of Nursing
University Hospitals of Cleveland
Clinical Associate Professor
Frances Payne Bolton School of Nursing
Case Western Reserve University
Cleveland, Ohio

LARK W. KIRK, Ph.D., R.N.
Assistant Professor and Faculty Associate for Research Development
Georgetown University
Washington, DC

HEIDI VONKOSS KROWCHUK, Ph.D., R.N.
Assistant Professor
Frances Payne Bolton School of Nursing
Case Western Reserve University
Cleveland, Ohio

SUSAN K. KUTZNER, Ph.D., R.N.
Associate Professor
School of Nursing
University of Texas Health Science Center at Houston
Houston, Texas

NANCY KLINE LEIDY, Ph.D., R.N.
Assistant Professor
College of Nursing
University of Arizona
Tucson, Arizona

MARTHA J. LENTZ, Ph.D., R.N.
Research Assistant Professor
School of Nursing
University of Washington
Seattle, Washington

MARIE L. LOBO, Ph.D., R.N.
Assistant Professor
College of Nursing
The Ohio State University
Columbus, Ohio

DEBORAH M. NADZAM, Ph.D., R.N.
Director of Nursing Research
Northwestern Memorial Hospital
Fellow, Center on Aging
McGaw Medical Center
Northwestern University
Chicago, Illinois

BEVERLY L. ROBERTS, Ph.D., R.N.
Assistant Professor
Frances Payne Bolton School of Nursing
Case Western Reserve University
Cleveland, Ohio

KATHLEEN ROSS-ALAOLMOLKI, Ph.D., R.N.
Assistant Professor
Frances Payne Bolton School of Nursing
Case Western Reserve University
Cleveland, Ohio

SAMUEL SCHULTZ II, Ph.D.
Associate Executive Director, Information Management
Hospital of the University of Pennsylvania
Philadelphia, Pennsylvania

JOANNE SABOL STEVENSON, Ph.D., F.A.A.N.
Professor
College of Nursing
The Ohio State University
Columbus, Ohio

ORA L. STRICKLAND, Ph.D., F.A.A.N.
Professor
School of Nursing
University of Maryland
Baltimore, Maryland

MARY ANN P. SWAIN, Ph.D.
Professor
School of Nursing
Associate Vice President for Academic Affairs
The University of Michigan
Ann Arbor, Michigan

BALDEO K. TANEJA, Ph.D.

Assistant Professor
Department of Mathematics and Statistics
Case Western Reserve University
Cleveland, Ohio

CAROLYN F. WALTZ, Ph.D., F.A.A.N.

Professor
School of Nursing
University of Maryland
Baltimore, Maryland

HARRIET H. WERLEY, Ph.D., F.A.A.N.

Distinguished Professor
School of Nursing
University of Wisconsin-Milwaukee
Milwaukee, Wisconsin

JERRY L. WESTON, SC.D., R.N.

Senior Research Manager
National Center for Health Services Research and
Health Care Technology Assessment
U.S. Department of Health and Human Services
Rockville, Maryland

ANN L. WHALL, Ph.D., F.A.A.N.

Professor
School of Nursing
The University of Michigan
Ann Arbor, Michigan

REG ARTHUR WILLIAMS, Ph.D., F.A.A.N.

Associate Professor
School of Nursing
The University of Michigan
Ann Arbor, Michigan

NANCY FUGATE WOODS, Ph.D., F.A.A.N.

Professor
School of Nursing
University of Washington
Seattle, Washington

STEPHEN J. ZYZANSKI, Ph.D.
Professor
Department of Family Medicine
School of Medicine
Case Western Reserve University
Cleveland, Ohio

PREFACE

With the continued expansion and sophistication of nursing and health research, it has become important, if not necessary, to address the role of statistics and quantitative methods as tools for research and knowledge development. In an effort to stimulate debate on these issues, the faculty of the Frances Payne Bolton School of Nursing at Case Western Reserve University sponsored a two-day multidisciplinary meeting: the *Invitational Conference on Statistics and Quantitative Methods*, held in Cleveland, on October 24-25, 1985. This book is a compilation of the edited papers and comments commissioned for that conference.

The formal introduction of statistics and quantitative methods in nursing and health research can be traced to the first graduate programs in nursing. Only recently, however, have issues pertaining to the integration of statistics, quantitative methods, and nursing been substantially addressed. Typical foci of debate center around graduate and doctoral curricula, qualifications for teaching statistics and quantitative methods in nursing, and the quantitative approach as excluding plurality in inquiry.

This debate about statistics and quantitative methods in nursing goes beyond curricular matters. It is directly related to the research enterprise in nursing, the standing of nursing research within the scientific community at large, and the scientific merit of nursing research. Above all, it is an interdisciplinary matter; the debate itself should not be conducted solely within nursing, but within a conglomerate of disciplines composed of nursing and other health sciences, theoretical and applied statistics, behavioral and social science, and computer and information science. There is a need for a systematic consideration of the integration of statistics and quantitative methods in the discipline of nursing concomitant with the rapid proliferation of doctoral programs in nursing and the growing scientific productivity within the discipline.

The *Invitational Conference on Statistics and Quantitative Methods in Nursing* and the present compilation of papers are intended to stimulate and contribute to this debate, as well as to offer initial direction for the further integration of quantitative science (i.e., statistics and quantitative methods, as defined by the American Statistical Association) in nursing research. This book, and the work and discussions it reflects, should not be seen as an endpoint, but rather as a point of departure for further work. Although the authors have addressed a number of crucial issues and provided many directives for the future, they also raise many questions and unresolved issues.

Following the structure of the conference, this book is organized in four parts. The first part includes comprehensive issues focused on the interface between statistics, quantitative methods, and nursing. It presents an overall frame of reference for thinking about statistics and quantitative methods in nursing research and education. Chapter 1, by Nadzam, Fitzpatrick, and Abraham, explores the demand for a quantitative nursing science for the profession and the discipline, and the educational and scientific nursing communities. They argue that statistics and quantitative methods are not only part of the syntactical structure of the discipline (i.e., the rules for determining what is valid about phenomena of concern), but also tools for explicating the discipline itself and for organizing its knowledge. In comments on this first chapter, Kirk proposes to monitor the evolution of the discipline of nursing along the four characteristics of a discipline. She offers a set of dimensions to aid in this monitoring process.

The issues raised in Chapter 1 and the accompanying comments are subsequently translated into curricular issues for integrating statistics and quantitative methods in nursing. The second chapter, co-authored by Abraham, Nadzam, and Fitzpatrick, addresses the issue of instructor qualifications and articulation of statistics curricula with the methodological, professional, and clinical components of nursing curricula. Ager, in comments on this chapter, emphasizes the need for prioritization of statistical content. Drawing upon his background as a psychologist, his teaching and consultation experience, and his ongoing collaborative efforts with nurse researchers, he offers suggestions for both master's and doctoral curricula.

Schultz (Chapter 3) reviews developments in information technology and statistical computing, and their pivotal role over the years in both the teaching and conduct of research in nursing. He stresses that great promises are held by innovative technology, in particular artifically intelligent scientific decision support systems, to research in nursing as well as knowledge development in nursing. Jane adds to this argument by elaborating on expert system models for statistical and methodological consultation.

The first part of the book concludes with a review of resources and structures necessary for the successful integration of statistics and quantitative methods in nursing education and research (Chapter 4). Stevenson uses a systems approach for this review, going from the needs of the individual researcher to the requirements for larger system resources and structures. In his comments, Cowling draws attention to the individual scientist as user and beneficiary of resources and structures. He argues that for these resources and structures to be effective, access channels for the individual nurse researcher should be developed to promote sustained scientific productivity.

The second part of this book is focused on the various speciality areas within nursing. Papers were commissioned from quantitative researchers within each specialty area with the specific request to prepare a contribution based on (1) what they perceived to be the more critical needs within their area, and how these needs could be best served through the conference and this book and (2) the availability (or nonavailability) of integrative reviews within their area that included quantitative dimensions.

Roberts (Chapter 5) reviews two years of publication of two prominent nursing research journals in an effort to identify and analyze trends in the use of statistics and quantitative methods used in medical-surgical nursing research. She identifies strengths and weaknesses and uses these to specify a set of methodological and statistical innovations for research in this specialty area. She stresses the need to adhere to normative rules for inquiry and analysis and the need to pursue the optimization of informativeness in research. In comments on this chapter, Leidy places Roberts' findings in a larger epistemological context and offers suggestions to enhance the methodological proficiency of research in medical-surgical nursing.

In Chapter 6, Lobo and Ross-Alaolmolki present a comprehensive overview of research on nursing care of children. They report on the frequency of use of research designs, measurement strategies, and statistical analyses, as well as on the ranges of sample sizes encountered in several volumes of a set of nursing journals. Guidelines for enhancing rigor and for expanding the empirical base in this speciality area are derived from the findings. Commenting on this chapter, Krowchuk links the Lobo and Ross-Alaolmolki findings and suggestions to recently observed trends in nursing research in general. She addresses implications of the current state of quantitative research in nursing care of children and offers additional suggestions for the future.

Lentz and Woods, in Chapter 7, build upon previous integrative reviews and summarize several methodological characteristics of inquiry in women's health. This is followed by methodological and statistical recommendations for studying issues central to women's health, such as transitions and dynamic processes. Arguing that women's health research is at a point where mere enumeration would be uninformative, the recommendations are presented innovatively by means of a description of an ongoing research project with extensive methodological and statistical demands. Kutzner comments that women's health may need to be placed within a nonsexist context of reproductive health. She also offers a few extensions and additions to shape the future of inquiry in the area.

Jones and Jones, in a chapter on psychiatric nursing research (Chapter 8), identify important aspects of researchers in this field, explicate the context within which this research was conducted and disseminated, and evaluate that appropriateness of use and sophistication level of statistical methods. This is done innovatively by means of a statistical evaluation of the literature of recent years. They present compelling data on the research context in psychiatric nursing and on the (in)ability of studies to detect significant differences in issues of statistical power, measurement, and design. Like so many of the other chapters in the second part of this book, their recommendations have implications that embrace all of nursing research. Williams extends the interpretation of the Jones and Jones findings to argue that research in psychiatric nursing may have been guided by relatively opportunistic matters. Pointing out that this might be good, given the state of the art in psychiatric as well as psychiatric-mental health nursing research, he offers recommendations to complement those of Jones and Jones.

In Chapter 9, Flynn builds upon recent reviews of research in community health nursing and proposes the elaboration model as a generic framework for data analysis in community health nursing research. The potential value of the model is illustrated with examples from the empirical literature in this specialty area, featuring studies that (unknowingly perhaps) applied the model and studies that did not apply it but revealed findings that could have been more informative if they had. The chapter concludes with some priority areas for research in community health nursing. Building upon Flynn's chapter, Goeppinger identifies five challenges that are pertinent to the field of community health nursing. She also argues the need to assess how statistics and quantitative methods can facilitate as well as inhibit progress toward meeting the challenges identified. Illustrations from her own research are used to clarify key points.

In Chapter 10, Whall, Booth, and Jirovec extend recent reviews addressing methodological issues in gerontological nursing research. They report on the prevalence of statistics in gerontological nursing research reports in two nursing journals over several decades. The trends noted are discussed in light of current educational opportunities in gerontological nursing, knowledge building in gerontological nursing research, and the relevance of the research reviewed to health care for older adults. Buckwalter comments on the Whall et al. findings as a point of departure for suggestions to increase both rigor and meaningfulness in gerontological nursing research. These suggestions are focused on the training of researchers for this area and on related empirical and statistical matters proper to the area.

In the final chapter of this part (Chapter 11), Halloran and Kiley, implying a general lack of accepted methodological and measurement strategies in research on nursing administration, focus their chapter on the use of a nursing diagnostic framework in the study of the organization and delivery of nursing services. After exploring nursing process as a referent of nursing care and critiquing existing methods for studying nursing care and work, Halloran and Kiley examine aspects of validity and reliability of measuring nursing process by means of nursing diagnosis. They link nursing diagnosis with nursing demand and resource allocation, thus demonstrating the feasibility of studying administrative issues in nursing within a context of cost. In her comments, Weston implies the need for some reservation and further work. She raises a number of important questions related to conceptualization and operationalization of demand, process, and outcome of nursing care.

The third part of this book is concerned with specific issues in the integration of quantitative science in nursing. Dennis (Chapter 12), pointing out the great potential held by multidisciplinary collaboration, presents structural descriptions of three collaborative models. This is followed by a discussion of methodological dilemmas inherent in, or at least amplified by, collaborative inquiry and by suggestions for addressing these dilemmas. Commenting on this chapter, Coulton extends Dennis' perspective on collaboration in research to collaboration in theory development. She stresses that it may be counterproductive to define excessively the boundaries of the different disciplines involved in interdisciplinary work.

Drawing upon her vast experience in the federal granting system, Harper (Chapter 13) presents advice on how to maximize the scientific merit of research grant applications and the likelihood of obtaining funding. Using a practical focus, she presents helpful information on the criteria for evaluation of proposals and reasons for disapproval. Zyzanski focuses his comments on the disapproval issues. He highlights two recurrently problematic areas: research design and computing and statistical analysis. His comments continue the practical focus adopted by Harper.

In Chapter 14, Grier and Foreman address the issue of effective presentation of scientific data. They provide guidelines for graphic, tabular, and statistical description of data sets. In her comments, Swain adds that the respective roles of graphics, tabulation, and statistical description should be placed within a larger epistemological context. This context should emphasize the importance of theory in the sophistication of analytic techniques, and it should be characterized by a commitment to replication and serial research.

Waltz and Strickland (Chapter 15) examine the measurement practices of nurse researchers undertaking studies of processes and outcomes in the literature. From this examination they identify issues and imperatives in the measurement of process and outcome variables that warrant attention if the reliability and validity of such studies are to be assured. Commenting on the chapter, Ferketich endorses the points made by Waltz and Strickland. She adds the measurement dilemma commonly faced by investigators of using either an established instrument with suboptimal match with the constructs of interest or a less validated one with great match. Her comments are focused on improving the expertise of researchers and on strategies for developing productive collaborative relationships between investigators and consultants in measurement and analysis.

Reflecting on more than a decade of teaching statistics in the health sciences, including nursing, Brogan presents a perspective of statisticians on nursing and nursing research (Chapter 16). She describes common views held by statisticians regarding the use of quantitative approaches in nursing. This is followed by a discussion of the teaching of statistics to students of nursing and how schools of nursing can collaborate with a (bio)statistics department within a university environment. She clarifies her views and concerns by considering issues related to women and quantitative science and concludes by calling for the licensing of statisticians. In his comments, Taneja, also a statistician, offers some suggestions regarding collaboration between researcher and statistician. As to education, he posits the need to balance demands for mathematical sophistication with the teaching of statistical thinking and proposes a three-step course sequence for achieving this in nursing.

The fourth and final part of this book features a summary chapter (Chapter 17) and comments on this chapter. Fitzpatrick, Abraham, and Nadzam stress the importance of intensifying the discussion initiated by this conference and book. This summary identifies four key issues: (1) delineation of the content of the discipline; (2) delineation of modes of inquiry for the discipline of nursing; (3) nature of the educational process, including professional and scientific socialization; and (4) research collaboration within the discipline. Strategies for the future conclude this chapter. Commenting on this final chapter, Werley offers helpful strategies to complement those identified by Fitzpatrick et al. She depicts an optimistic view on progress in nursing science.

As we noted earlier, this book and the *Invitational Conference on Statistics and Quantitative Methods in Nursing* on which it is based are proposed as a beginning, not an end point. The aim was to assess the past and present of quantitative science in nursing so as to guide future developments. The work should serve as a synthesis for those committed to the further expansion and sophistication of nursing science.

We wish to conclude this preface chapter by recognizing the contributions and support of several people. The *Invitational Conference on Statistics and Quantitative Methods in Nursing* was made possible by the financial support of the Frances Payne Bolton School of Nursing at Case Western Reserve University. The support of the administration of the university is recognized. The many participants of the conference, who provided additional depth to the contributions of the speakers and authors, deserve recognition. Also, we want to emphasize the professional wisdom of Dudley R. Kay, former Publisher and Department Head of Nursing and Allied Health at W. B. Saunders Company, who supported the publication of this book. We have learned that it is rather uncommon among publishers to be concerned primarily with the advancement of the discipline of nursing. We also wish to acknowledge the editorial assistance of C. Valerie Rice. Finally, we deeply thank Sabrina Harris for her text processing support and her diligence in moving this book through its several versions.

IVO L. ABRAHAM, Ph.D., R.N.
DEBORAH M. NADZAM, Ph.D., R.N.
JOYCE J. FITZPATRICK, Ph.D, F.A.A.N.

CONTENTS

PART 2

Quantitative Science in Nursing Research

PART 3

Issues in the Integration of Nursing and Quantitative Science

PART 4

Conclusion and Summary

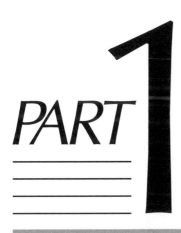

PART 1

Interfacing Nursing and Quantitative Science

1

Statistics, Quantitative Methods, and the Discipline of Nursing

DEBORAH M. NADZAM, Ph.D., R.N.
JOYCE J. FITZPATRICK, Ph.D., F.A.A.N.
IVO L. ABRAHAM, Ph.D., R.N.

Characteristics of a Discipline
The Status of Nursing as a Discipline
The Interface Between Nursing and Statistics
Comment: Quantitative Science and the Evolution of the Discipline

Ellis (1984) stated that the body of knowledge of the field of nursing can be organized according to the three major activities for which nurses have responsibility: nursing practice, nursing education, and nursing inquiry. Nursing practice is concerned with the *use* of knowledge and has as its goal, "beneficence for patients" (Ellis, 1984). Nursing education focuses on the *transmission* and *acquisition* of knowledge, with a goal of preparing practitioners, educators, administrators, and scholars. Nursing inquiry is concerned with the *organization* and *development* of knowledge. The second and third activities, nursing education and nursing inquiry, are the focus of this book. This chapter focuses on the third activity, nursing inquiry. Specifically, we propose two major areas of interface between the discipline of nursing and statistics and quantitative methods: (1) the role of statistics and quantitative methods as part of the syntactical structure of the discipline; and (2) their role in further explicating the discipline as a whole. As an introduction, we first review the status of nursing as a discipline.

Characteristics of a Discipline

A discipline is defined as a distinct way of knowing or learning that involves research (Foshay, 1961). Foshay (1961) identified four characteristics of a discipline that define its separateness and uniqueness from other disciplines: domain, rules for inquiry, history, and output.

The domain of a discipline, also referred to as the *conceptual structure* by Schwab (1962), is the content or subject matter of interest to members of the discipline. It identifies the phenomena about which truth is sought and is expected to change as a result of inquiry. The domain is structured and bound by the unique perspective of the discipline, which guides investigators and leads them to inquiry.

The rules for inquiry are the agreed-upon methods for determining what is valid about the phenomena. Schwab (1962) referred to these rules as the *syntactical structure*. The syntax is the process through which members of the discipline determine what is true or almost true.

History, the third characteristic of a discipline, shapes both the domain and the rules for inquiry. A review of where the field of inquiry has been and is not, determines the kinds of questions asked in future research. There is evidence of building upon past research.

The fourth characteristic is output, which includes the knowledge discovered through research. It may be in the form of facts, statements, or theory. Both history and output help to organize the knowledge about the domain developed through the rules of inquiry (syntax).

The Status of Nursing as a Discipline

The four characteristics of a discipline as identified by Foshay (1961) are now reviewed from a nursing perspective, to describe more clearly the status of the discipline of nursing. Of the four characteristics of a discipline, nurse scholars have most clearly identified its domain. Several nursing theorists have agreed that the concepts of interest to nursing as a field of inquiry are person, environment, health, and nursing (Chinn, 1983; Fawcett, 1984; Fitzpatrick & Whall, 1983; Flaskerud & Halloran, 1980; Gortner, 1983; Kim, 1983). It is important to point out that, although there is consensus about these four concepts, there is agreement only on the terms themselves, not on the meaning of the four concepts (Ellis, 1982). Furthermore, the identification of *concepts* does not fully describe the phenomena of interest to nurses. Concepts are mental pictures or ideas; phenomena are observables and are measurable. Donaldson and Crowley (1977) also have identified three major themes of interest that shape the perspective of the discipline of nursing. The three themes are concerned with relationships between the four preceding concepts: relationships between (1) person and environment; (2) person and health; and (3) person, health, and nursing actions. Although the conceptual structure of nursing has developed significantly over the past 20 years and a metaparadigm is apparent (Fawcett, 1984), continued specification is essential.

Of the four characteristics, the syntactical structure of the discipline of nursing is least well defined. Carper (1975) identified four patterns of knowing in nursing empirics, nursing aesthetics, ethics, and synoetics—each of which may call for different modes of inquiry. Nurse theorists agree on the different patterns of knowing (Carper, 1975; Donaldson & Crowley, 1978; Duffy, 1985; Ellis, 1984; Fawcett, 1984; Gortner, 1983; Munhall, 1982) and agree on the need for multiple modes of inquiry. At this time the classical scientific approach of logical positivism has received considerable support by nurse scholars. But this approach is applicable only to empirical questions posed by nurses. Ethical questions may call for philosophical inquiry and perhaps historical inquiry. Aesthetics and synoetics are being researched using qualitative and phenomenological approaches (Fawcett,

1984; Oiler, 1982; Omery, 1983). Fawcett (1984) does not rule out the possible use of empirical methods in researching ethics, aesthetics, and synoetics. Nurse scholars generally agree, however, that studying holistic human beings cannot be achieved solely through empirics. Hence, the syntactical structure of nursing as a discipline has not been clearly identified. There is only beginning agreement that one mode of inquiry is not sufficient.

The history of nursing is a long one; however, the history of formal nursing research is relatively recent. This is as troubling as the noted lack of structure of the knowledge discovered. There is little evidence in nursing research of organization, replication, and building upon past studies. Only recently has emphasis been placed upon the need to replicate studies. Consequently, the discipline has not defined its domain and rules as quickly as it might have. However, there have been some positive gains from reviewing the history. One result worthy of note has been identification of the need for more clinical research; that is, research focused on clients rather than on nurses. In 1977, Gortner pointed out that most published research in nursing was concerned with nurses themselves. There has been a more concerted effort in recent years to distinguish among nursing research, research on the profession, and research on education (Bloch, 1982). History, as a characteristic of a discipline, has begun to affect the development of research within the discipline.

Finally, nursing inquiry has resulted in significant output. However, this has been primarily through individuals' efforts, with less systematic regard for the larger domain of nursing or reference to conceptual frameworks for nursing. The limited output of nursing research is still a reflection of the state of the other three characteristics of a discipline. Until there is greater consensus about domain and rules and until past research findings and implications are built upon, the knowledge discovered through nursing inquiry will continue to be scattered and less structured than what is desired.

The Interface Between Nursing and Statistics

Given the current status of the discipline of nursing, how do statistics and quantitative methods interface with it? To identify this interface, definitions of statistics and quantitative methods are now offered. Noether (1971) quotes a U.S. Civil Service Commission document to define statistics as "the science of collection, classification, and measured evaluation of facts as a basis for inference. It is a body of techniques for acquiring accurate knowledge from incomplete information; a scientific system for the collection, organization, analysis, interpretation and presentation of information which can be stated in numerical form" (p. 1). We must distinguish quantitative methods from quantitative *research*. Quantitative research most often refers to experimental design, the empiricist approach, and deductive reasoning. Quantitative methods are statistical and mathematical approaches to analyzing data, regardless of the type or design of the study.

Considering these definitions of statistics and quantitative methods, and following the review of the status of nursing as a discipline, two areas of interface are apparent: (1) the role of statistics and quantitative methods as part of the syntactical structure of the discipline and (2) the role of statistics and quantitative methods in further explicating the discipline as a whole. These two areas are discussed in greater detail.

To understand the role of statistics and quantitative methods as part of the syntactical structure, we reemphasize the difference between quantitative methods and quantitative research. The syntactical structure speaks to the type of research, or theory-generating approach, as well as to methods for determining what is valid or not valid about the phenomena of interest. Quantitative methods and statistics are not theory-generating approaches. Rather, they are modes for analyzing data gathered from any of the theory-generating approaches. Thus, in accordance with Noether's (1971) definition of statistics, any information that can be stated in numerical form is amenable to statistical application.

The question now becomes: what information can be stated in numerical form? By using one or more of the four levels of numerical scales—nominal, ordinal, interval, and ratio—most information can be stated in numbers. Thus, most information, or data, is amenable to statistical analysis of some type. Stating information in interval and ratio levels is preferred. Abdellah and Levine (1965) outline several advantages of these two quantitative, or measurement, scales, including greater accuracy, objectivity, sensitivity, and versatility. Data on the interval and ratio levels can be subjected to several statistical procedures. To list these is beyond the scope of this chapter; the reader is referred to the numerous textbooks on statistical inference. It is sufficient to note that the quantitative methods available for application are numerous and specific to the kinds of questions being asked. The artistry in application of these methods rests in researchers' ability to choose knowledgeably the appropriate method of analysis, to attend carefully to interpretation of findings, and to recognize limitations when they exist.

The role of statistics and quantitative methods must be enhanced beyond the elementary utilization currently found in nursing research. One way to achieve enhancement is to employ multivariate statistical techniques first to quantify and then to examine qualitative data. Qualitative data can be converted to numbers via the classification scales of nominal and ordinal levels, thus making these data open to statistical analysis.

Realizing that qualitative researchers will claim loss of sensitivity and precision if data are quantified, it becomes essential to state the advantages and gains to be made from this quantification process. The several multi-variate statistical techniques provide processes for testing classification and for identifying patterns and profiles of phenomena being researched. Discriminant function analysis, principal-components analysis, factor analysis, cluster analysis, and multivariate analysis of variance are adjunct methods for describing qualitative data (adjunct to the researchers' expert view and description provided through word symbols). These multivariate techniques have been severely underutilized in nursing research. Granted, results of statistically analyzing quantified qualitative data are descriptive and explanatory; however, this method may stimulate the generation of testable hypotheses, or identify mechanisms for measuring the particular phenomena on ratio and interval levels. These results may lead to improved measurement, as well as to increased rigor.

Statistics and quantitative methods are tools for analyzing the data obtained from any kind of theory-generating approach and are a part of the syntactical structure of the discipline of nursing. Therefore, nurse researchers must familiarize themselves with various statistical methods, beyond the elementary rules for application.

Here we outline four immediate suggestions for nurse researchers who are interested in increasing the rigor of their studies. These suggestions pertain to sampling theory, principles of experimental design, establishment of confidence intervals, and validation of assumptions. These suggestions are more than suggestions to the statistician; they are based on proven mathematical and statistical theory. Although we are not asking nurses to be statisticians (or are we?), attention to these suggestions would certainly increase the rigor of nursing research and must be incorporated into the discipline's syntactical structure.

The first suggestion follows observation of constant concern over, and often erroneous determination of, sample size. This problem can be addressed through the institution of pilot studies and application of knowledge derived from sampling theory. Sampling theory provides mechanisms for random selection of elements from one group, like groups, or unlike groups. More important, sampling theory provides for mathematical determination of the establishment of the N needed to estimate the population. Increased application of these statistically sound techniques would provide rationale for the chosen sample size, increase rigor, and be more efficient in knowledge generation.

The second suggestion is recommended adherence to a set of principles for experimental design. Fisher (1947) advocated the importance of attending to randomization, replication, and error control when designing an experiment. Random assignment of elements to treatment cells, replication or several runs of treatments, and control of errors through blocking all serve to increase independence of error, reduce the error, and provide a more valid estimate of this error. Although these principles sound elementary to those familiar with them, the fact remains that they are not well followed in nursing research, perhaps because the theory supporting each one is not taught or because the educational level is just now being heightened.

The third and fourth suggestions related to statistical inference are infrequently referred to in reports of nursing research. The establishment of confidence intervals and the validation of assumptions serve to strengthen inferences made. Confidence intervals are established to determine the generalizability and predictive power of findings. Yet they are only as confident as the assumptions are valid; the usual assumptions being independence of errors, normal distribution of errors, and constant variance. Rarely in published nursing research is there evidence of residual analysis, the ·process by which assumptions are checked and confidence intervals are made meaningful.

The preceding four suggestions are offered only to highlight "rules" expected to be followed by statisticians. The power and credulence of research is suspect if even basics are overlooked. As scholars, we shape the discipline of nursing and should expect a sophisticated approach to inquiry. Advanced use of statistics and quantitative methods must become part of the syntactical structure of the discipline of nursing.

The second major area of interface between statistics and quantitative methods and the discipline of nursing is concerned with how the former can advance the latter. The effect of statistics and quantitative methods on the discipline as a whole rests with points made in the preceding discussion. Increased knowledge and sophisticated application of advanced statistical techniques will enable researchers to define the domain more clearly, will offer methods for reviewing past research, will assist with the organization of knowledge, and will most certainly provide for more meaningful output.

Multivariate techniques can enable researchers to describe phenomena and lead to reliable and valid measurement techniques. Members of the discipline will then be able to move from exploratory and descriptive research to empirical research utilizing principles of experimental design and will be able to test interventions and demonstrate causal relationships.

The application of other statistical methods must also be incorporated into the syntactical structure of the nursing discipline. Meta-analysis can facilitate the summary and synthesis of many research efforts, leading to identification of trends and suggestions for future research. Nonparametric methods are grossly underutilized, yet they provide a means for analyzing ordinal data. They also can be used with interval and ratio data when assumptions underlying parametric tests are violated—not an uncommon characteristic of the data we tend to collect in nursing and health research. Time series analysis can be applied to longitudinal studies of the effects of specific nursing interventions. This quantitative method provides for the ability to analyze change over time, a process that could strengthen inferences of causality. Expanded understanding and application of analysis of variance techniques is needed, including complex factorial designs and block designs. These proposed statistical applications certainly are not all-inclusive. Obviously, several other quantitative methods available.

In summary, in this chapter we have outlined the status of the discipline of nursing and the interface of nursing, statistics, and quantitative methods. To advance the discipline as a whole, nurse scholars must increase their own sophistication with statistics and quantitative methods. In response to the consulting statistician (or perhaps even the disbelieving nurse researcher), who may ask why nurse scholars must grasp this knowledge rather than hire a consultant, we offer two quotes. The first, from Box, Hunter, and Hunter's *Statistics for Experimenters* (1978), reminds us to consider our own perspective when using statistics:

Experimenters, when you are doing "statistics" do not forget what you know about your subject-matter field! Statistical techniques are most effective when combined with appropriate subject-matter knowledge. The methods are an important adjunct to, not a replacement for the natural skill of the experimenter. [p. 15]

The second quote, from Marriot's *The Interpretation of Multiple Observations* (1974), cautions against blind faith in numbers and disregard for expert knowledge:

If the results disagree with informed opinion, do not admit a simple logical interpretation, and do not show up clearly in a graphical presentation, they are probably wrong. There is no magic about numerical methods, and [there are] many ways in which they can break down. They are a valuable aid to the interpretation of data, not sausage machines automatically transforming bodies of numbers into packets of scientific fact. [p. 89]

We say the discipline of nursing has a unique perspective and asks certain questions of certain phenomena. We must be prepared to explain, describe, and analyze the phenomena of interest from this perspective. The skilled and artful application of statistics and quantitative methods thus becomes an attribute of nurse researchers.

REFERENCES

Abdellah, F. G., & Levine, E. (1965). *Better patient care through nursing research*. New York: Macmillan.

Bloch, D. (1982). A conceptualization of nursing research and nursing science. In McCloskey, J. C. & Grace, H. K. (Eds.), *Current issues in nursing*. Worcester, MA: Blackwell Scientific.

Box, G. E. R., Hunter, W. G., & Hunter, J. S. (1978). *Statistics for experimenters: An introduction to design, data analysis and model building*. New York: Wiley.

Carper, B. A. (1975). *Fundamental patterns of knowing in nursing*. Unpublished Ph.D. Dissertation, Teachers College, Columbia University, New York.

Chinn, P. L. (1983). Nursing theory development: Where we have been and where we are going. In N. L. Chaska (Ed.), *The nursing profession: A time to speak*. New York: McGraw-Hill.

Donaldson, S. K., & Crowley, D. M. (1978). Discipline of nursing: Structure and relationship to practice. *Nursing Outlook, 26,* 113–120.

Duffy, M. E. (1985). Designing nursing research: The qualitative–quantitative debate. *Journal of Advanced Nursing, 10,* 225–232.

Ellis, R. (1982). Conceptual issues in nursing. *Nursing Outlook, 30,* 406–410.

Ellis, R. (1984). Nursing knowledge development. *Proceedings of doctoral forum on doctoral education in nursing: Epistemological strategies in nursing.* Denver: University of Colorado School of Nursing.

Fawcett, J. (1984). Hallmarks of success in nursing research. *Advances in Nursing Science, 7,* 1–10.

Fisher, R. A. (1947). *The design of experiments.* London: Oliver & Boyd.

Fitzpatrick J. J., & Whall, A. (Eds.) (1983). *Conceptual models of nursing: Analysis and application.* Bowie, MD: Brady.

Flaskerud, J. H., & Halloran, E. J. (1980). Areas of agreement in nursing theory development. *Advances in Nursing Science, 3*(1), 1–7.

Foshay, A. W. (1961). *Knowledge and structure of the discipline.* Paper presented at "The Nature of Knowledge Conference," University of Wisconsin, Madison, WI.

Gortner, S. (1983). The history and philosophy of nursing research. *Advances in Nursing Science, 6,* 2–8.

Kim, S. H. (1983). *The nature of theoretical thinking in nursing.* Norwalk, CT: Appleton-Century-Crofts.

Marriot, F. H. C. (1974). *The interpretation of multiple observations.* Orlando, FL: Academic.

Munhall, P. L. (1982). Nursing philosophy and nursing research: In apposition or opposition? *Nursing Research, 31,* 176–181.

Noether, G. (1971). *Introduction to statistics.* Boston: Houghton Mifflin.

Oiler, C. (1982). The phenomenological approach to nursing research. *Nursing Research, 31,* 78–81.

Omery, A. (1983). Phenomenology: A method for nursing research. *Advances in Nursing Science, 5,* 49–63.

Schwab, J. J. (1962). The concept of the structure of a discipline. *The Education Record, 43,* 197–205.

Comment

Quantitative Science and the Evolution of the Discipline

LARK W. KIRK, Ph.D., R.N.

The preceding chapter includes a wealth of provocative ideas for those concerned with the efficiency and reliability of knowledge development and organization in nursing. The authors present a justified and well-documented perspective on the integration of statistics and quantitative methods in nursing. The ideas and assertions are well supported by both reason and fact. It is important to emphasize and examine at least a few of the core ideas of that chapter.

The main thesis of the chapter is that the process of knowledge development in nursing will be enhanced by merging (1) the evolving understanding of nursing as an academic discipline or field of inquiry with (2) the more classic and longstanding recognition of the key role of statistics and quantitative methods within all disciplines concerned with empirical referents and measurement. This raises the question as to how progress in the evolution of nursing can be monitored.

Following Foshay (1961), the authors outlined four characteristics of a discipline. These characteristics can be translated into four dimensions along which we can monitor the evolution of nursing as a scientific discipline. The first proposed dimension, "domain specification," refers to the extent to which nursing, through the knowledge it has gained, affirms itself as a scientific discipline with distinct boundaries. "Clarity and completeness of rules or syntax" is the second dimension. It is concerned with the extent to which nursing, in its effort to consolidate itself as a scientific discipline, elucidates the format and context of its scientific activities. The third dimension is "comprehension of and connection to historical background"; it emphasizes the importance of placing the evolution of nursing science within a historical context, so as to understand the present and project the future. The final dimension, "output of research programs," is defined as the degree to which the research output exhibits coherence and organization. It should be pointed out that monitoring the discipline of nursing along these dimensions implies a logical positivist view of science.

In the preceding chapter, statistics and quantitative methods are argued to be part of the syntactical structure of the discipline, but they are also proposed as tools to aid in explicating the discipline and achieving reorganization of knowledge. This is a most innovative perspective and aids in clarifying the basis for an interdisciplinary agreement on processes for deciding what is scientifically valid. When the knowledge gains in nursing have attained the necessary level and general progress (as defined earlier), it will indeed be due to gains dependent in part upon lucid and well-chosen statistical and quantitative approaches. Without such agreement the collective work of the nursing discipline as a community of discoursers (King & Brownell, 1966) cannot proceed. The firm position offered in the chapter on the importance of quantitative science holds promise for aiding the acceptance of nursing as a discipline among colleagues in other fields, most notably in those fields in which empirical inquiry and corresponding statistical approaches have enjoyed a longer tradition.

In closing, although the nursing literature demonstrates a rapidly growing number of papers providing a philosophical or historical treatment of knowledge development and knowledge organization (e.g., Brooks & Kleine-Kracht, 1983; Carper, 1978; Conway, 1985; Gorenberg, 1983; Gortner & Nahm, 1977; Hinshaw, 1979; Loomis, 1985; Silva & Rothbart, 1984; Smith, 1984; Thompson, 1985), the preceding chapter is distinguished by approaching these topics on a quantitative scientific basis.

REFERENCES

Brooks, J. A., & Kleine-Kracht, A. E. (1983). Evolution of a definition of nursing. *Advances in Nursing Science, 5*(1), 51–85.

Carper, B. A. (1978). Fundamental patterns of knowing in nursing. *Advances in Nursing Science, 1*(1), 13–23.

Conway, M. E. (1985). Toward greater specificity in defining nursing's meta-paradigm. *Advances in Nursing Science, 7*(4), 73–81.

Foshay, A. W. (1961). *Knowledge and structure of the discipline.* Paper presented at "The Nature of Knowledge Conference," University of Wisconsin–Madison, WI.

Gorenberg, B. (1983). The research tradition in nursing: An emerging issue. *Nursing Research, 32,* 347–349.

Gortner, S. R., & Nahm, H. (1977). An overview of nursing research in the United States. *Nursing Research, 26,* 10–33.

Hinshaw, A. S. (1979). Theoretical substruction: An assessment process. *Western Journal of Nursing Research, 1,* 319–324.

King, A. R., & Brownell, J. A. (1966). *The curriculum and the discipline of knowledge: A theory of curriculum practice.* New York: Wiley.

Loomis, M. E. (1985). Emerging content in nursing: An analysis of dissertation abstracts and titles 1976-1982. *Nursing Research, 34,* 113–119.

Silva, M. C., & Rothbart, D. (1984). An analysis of changing trends in philosophies of science on nursing theory development and testing. *Advances in Nursing Science, 6*(2), 1–13.

Smith, M. C. (1984). Research methodology: Epistemologic considerations. *Image: The Journal of Nursing Scholarship, 16*(2), 42–46.

Thompson, J. L. (1985). Practical discourse in nursing: Going beyond empiricism and historicism. *Advances in Nursing Science, 7*(4), 59–71.

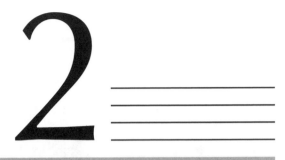

Statistics in Nursing Curricula

IVO L. ABRAHAM, Ph.D., R.N.
DEBORAH M. NADZAM, Ph.D., R.N.
JOYCE J. FITZPATRICK, Ph.D., F.A.A.N.

This chapter is concerned with issues in the development of curricula for teaching statistics in nursing education. The proposed perspective is that scholars and scientists should be highly adept at invoking tools and aids that may assist them in the development and implementation of their research and that their ability to do so characterizes them as such (Fitzpatrick & Abraham, 1987). Mastery of sophisticated statistical applications, grounded in an adequate understanding of supporting theory, is a basic scientific skill in nursing.

The promotion of the teaching of statistics in nursing is determined by a variety of factors. These pertain to the student population served, the availability and qualifications of faculty, the academic environment, and specific issues in statistics and quantitative science. In this chapter we review determinants of teaching statistics in academic nursing and discuss curricular issues. This review and discussion then serve as the basis for formulating a set of recommendations.

This chapter, with its focus on scientists and scholars, is geared toward master's and doctoral education in nursing. Furthermore, it is presumed that, at the master's level, research is an integral component of the curriculum and that research prevails at the doctoral (academic research doctorate) level.

We purposely refrain from developing a model curriculum for teaching statistics in nursing, and even from a prescriptive listing of topics to be covered, because decisions about the integration of statistics into curricula are determined by many more factors than just content. Instead we focus on curricular goals related to qualities and competencies; the emphasis is therefore on developing a frame of reference for the design and implementation of statistical curricula in nursing.

Statistics and Quantitative Science in Nursing

STUDENTS

The success of any teaching program is in part determined by the extent to which the students view the content as relevant to current and future personal objectives. There is evidence that students in nursing hold coursework in quantitative science in low regard. Passos and Stallings (1973) taught measurement and statistics to sophomore nursing students and found that 40% of the students did not favor the course, with most of the remaining students being undecided about its relevance. Brogan (1980a, 1982) observed that master's students in nursing appreciate research courses more than statistics courses. She also found that coursework in research and statistics did not produce significant changes in students' interest in research as part of their career. Thus, interest in quantitative science among students in nursing may be equivocal at best.

Abraham (1984) offered traditional female socialization patterns as a partial explanation for this limited interest. From early childhood on, women are generally socialized to eschew mathematics, exact sciences, technology, and more recently, computers. Languages, social science, and behavioral science are encouraged instead. This results in a paradoxical situation: Fewer women are advised to commit themselves to quantitatively oriented pursuits and careers (in casu, scientist), yet those who are committed to these pursuits suffer from the relative neglect of mathematics and sciences in American high school curricula. The (societally unjustified) end product is often a woman of great intelligence, with great potential as a scientist, but with limited quantitative and empirical skills.

It is not uncommon to find a wide discrepancy in quantitative skills among students entering master's and, in particular, doctoral programs (most often reflected in their Quantitative Graduate Records Examination scores as well). Only a very small minority have a calculus background. More have a background in intermediate algebra, but they are not necessarily in the majority. It is indeed unfortunate that graduate programs in nursing are faced with applicants and students whose reason for arriving at a positive number when multiplying two negative numbers is that the minuses cancel each other.

Although no empirical evidence is available, it appears that, in general, students in nursing programs tend to be mathematically below par when compared with their counterparts in many other disciplines. Yet simultaneously they are confronted with the same demands of scientific rigor and credibility as those faced by their counterparts with better-developed quantitative skills.

FACULTY

The teaching of statistics in schools of nursing is complicated by the relative unavailability of credentialed faculty to teach such courses at the master's and doctoral level—that is, faculty "with a formal degree or doctoral minor in (applied) statistics, with sufficient expertise, and/or with scientific recognition (publications and juried presentations)" (Abraham, 1984, p. 3). Hence, many schools recruit nonnursing faculty to teach these courses (most often behavioral and social scientists with an applied statistics background); in other schools students take service courses offered by the university's statistics department.

Some data are available regarding in-house instructors in medicine and nursing. From a survey of American and Canadian medical schools, Colton (1975) developed the following profile. Most biostatistics instructors in medical schools are males (93%) under age 40 (50%) with a nonmedical doctorate (66% had either a Ph.D., Sc.D., Ed.D., or Dr.P.H.; 18% had an M.D.; also, 15% had bachelor's or master's degrees). Formal graduate education was usually obtained in either biostatistics (35%), statistics (25%), or mathematics (13%); other fields included biomathematics, economics, psychology, and sociology. Remarkably, 8% had no formal training in statistics or quantitative science.

Shelton (1979) surveyed baccalaureate nursing programs that have research methods and statistics courses as degree requirements. Whereas research courses were most often taught by nursing faculty, only 8% of the schools had their own faculty teach statistics courses (5% in colleges, 19% in universities). Most often statistics was taught by behavioral or social scientists. These findings pertain to baccalaureate education in nursing; no systematic data are available on master's and doctoral education. Anecdotal evidence, however, suggests a similar pattern.

The responsibilities of statistics instructors in schools of nursing are seldom limited to teaching and research. In many cases, they are the (informally or formally appointed) consultant and resource person, often for matters far exceeding statistics: design, instrument development, computing (including equipment management), and proposal development.

ACADEMIC ENVIRONMENT

Teaching statistics may be hampered further if it occurs in an environment with limited scientific credibility. If statistics is indeed to serve as a tool for scientific progress, then it is imperative that scientific activity be evidenced within the school of nursing. Realistically, however, although there are many (often self-proclaimed) researchers in nursing, there are few centers of scientific excellence; their percentage of the total number of master's and doctoral programs is very small. Consequently, many nursing students are taught statistics and quantitative science. A sizable proportion of these students must do an empirical thesis or dissertation, but few have sufficiently trained instructors to learn how to use statistics most efficiently and how to apply it so that its scientific relevance is maximized.

STATISTICS AND QUANTITATIVE SCIENCE

What type of statistics should be taught in academic nursing programs, and consequently, what knowledge and application skills are expected of students? Within statistics, a distinction between mathematical and applied statistics usually is made, with the latter category being of most relevance to scientists in the different disciplines. Under ideal conditions, applied statistics should refer to the application of statistical procedures to the study of specific discipline-related phenomena so as to aid in arriving at sound scientific inferences. Where indicated, this includes the refinement of mathematical statistical procedures to the specifics of scientific inquiry in a given discipline. Note that with its emphasis on application and creative manipulation, applied statistics requires a relatively high level of cognitive functioning.

In nursing and a few other disciplines, a third type of statistics is not uncommon, namely, watered-down statistics, in which an understanding of concepts and theory is not required, the focus instead being on the (flawless) identification and application of presumably appropriate techniques. An example might go as follows: "I have two groups. My dependent variable is at the interval level, so I do a t-test and hope the p is smaller than .05." Little or no consideration is given to statistical assumptions to be met, the alternative of nonparametric procedures, or statistical power—let alone advanced issues such as effect size, measures of association, and explained variance.

Courses in watered-down statistics tend to emphasize the mastery of a limited number of crucial concepts (levels of measurement, alpha level, t-test, F-test, correlation). This then serves as the basis for teaching a set of quasi-algorithmic rules for selecting statistical procedures (see, for example, the preceding t-test example). The implicit or explicit goal of instruction, often encountered in one form or another in course syllabuses, is to be able to select an appropriate statistical test for answering the research question asked.

The matter is further complicated by the adoption of traditional perspectives on what statisticians do. Especially among master's students, the purpose of statistics is viewed to be description (by means of descriptive statistics) and general inference (by means of procedures for hypothesis testing), with correlation being the alternative when a noncomparative design is used. Doctoral students tend to develop broader perspectives, including multiple regression and complex analysis of variance models. Only a few programs offer multivariate procedures, but they seldom treat topics specific to nursing and health research (such as the measurement of change, exploratory data analysis, censored data sets, and statistical consultation skills). Again, in many instances, the teaching is limited to a functional "cookbook" approach.

Although multivariate statistics has found its way into some doctoral programs in nursing, there appears to be confusion about what procedures fall in this category. Recent textbooks illustrate the problem. Volicer (1984) published a text entitled *Multivarate Statistics for Nursing Research* that is minimally concerned with multivariate statistics. It deals extensively with *t*-tests, chi-square tests, regression and correlation, multiple regression, and analysis of variance models. Only one chapter, just 11 pages long (out of more than 300), deals with multivariate statistics and covers factor analysis and discriminant analysis. The level of sophistication of this chapter should be subject to debate. A text by Shelley (1984) focuses upon quantitative research methods but has several chapters on statistical procedures. Multivariate statistics is given minimal consideration, even though the book is targeted for intermediate and advanced students.

Multivariate statistics should be fully integrated into the curricula of doctoral programs in nursing and should be made a degree requirement. This is predicated on the fact that the phenomena of concern in nursing are complex and involve many interrelated variables. Paradigms for multivariable inquiry and procedures for their statistical analysis need to be taught.

Curricular Issues

The successful implementation of statistics courses in nursing curricula is not contingent solely upon the consideration of the factors and issues identified earlier. Curricular issues must also be addressed: mathematical sophistication of the course, statistical procedures to be included, and sequencing of content.

MATHEMATICAL SOPHISTICATION

As mentioned earlier, few master's and doctoral students in nursing have had calculus, and the percentage of students with a knowledge of even algebra and geometry is often low. A curriculum with heavy emphasis on mathematical inference is understood only by the better-prepared students. Nonetheless, can we teach students to make accurate and detailed estimations, judgments, and decisions, using the most appropriate statistical techniques at their disposition? The key is probably the extent to which arithmetic, theory, and application are balanced. With the wide availability of computer facilities for statistical inference it is no longer necessary to teach computational formulas and their proofs and to require their memorization. Instead, teaching students the elements of a formula and the reasoning underlying their integration into this formula is indicated, the goal being an adequate understanding of the "operations" of a given test. Further, students should be taught that there is more to statistics than the application of quasi-algorithmic rules.

CONTENT

It is important to deemphasize hypothesis testing and correlational analysis as the primary purpose of statistics. Instead, it should be stressed continuously that statistical procedures exist for a variety of applications, from testing differences to modeling relationships among variables, classifying subjects, reducing complexity, and exploring structure. In addition, students need to be taught that there is no direct link between research questions and statistical method and that the only existing direct link in statistics is between data and test alternatives (plural emphasized). Hence, it is imperative to teach students to familiarize themselves with their sample data through graphical visualization and tabular presentation, to investigate whether statistical assumptions have been met, and to consider the application of additional tests so as to maximize the informativeness of inferences made.

Especially in doctoral education, a major proportion of statistics courses should deal with advanced statistical procedures. Multivariate statistics is a necessity because of the phenomena of concern in nursing and should be a degree requirement. However, the specifics of nursing research warrant the inclusion of several other topics. First, since much research in nursing is concerned with change over time, coursework should include the measurement of change, from simple pre- and postanalysis to time series analysis, time profile analysis, and stochastic models such as Markov chains. Second, since nursing research is most often conducted under suboptimal conditions, with restricted randomization and (high) subject attrition, students should be taught, respectively, the statistical analysis of research in field settings and the management of incomplete or censored data sets. Finally, because many doctorally prepared nurse researchers are faced with demands for statistical experience, attention should be devoted to the development of consultation skills.

Finally, some statistical topics cut across educational levels and should be considered for inclusion to the extent appropriate for a given level. These are probability, uncertainty in judgment, statistical inference, and the relationships among these concepts; statistical interaction; theory of and procedures for statistical power analysis; statistical consequences of randomized, matched, and cohort subsamples; serial testing and the inflated probability of Type I errors; the measurement of effect size as a complement to hypothesis testing; and the (mis)use of measures of explained variance.

SEQUENCING OF CONTENT

In her description of the statistics sequence in the Master of Nursing program at Emory University, Brogan (1980a, 1980b) made a case for teaching nonparametric statistics before introducing parametric procedures. Nonparametrics "follow logically from the concept of probability and appear, intuitively, to be reasonable ways to analyze data" (Brogan, 1980b, p. 103) and "are easily and quickly calculated, allowing students time to become familiar with statistics" (Brogan, 1980b, p. 104). Further, Brogan (1980a) argued that most research projects in nursing yield data bases that do not meet statistical assumptions for parametric techniques and therefore should be analyzed using distribution-free methods. The didactic relevance of teaching nonparametics first has also been demonstrated in liberal arts education (Lefkon, Fletcher, & Derderian, 1976).

Brogan's stand in favor of nonparametrics finds little support in nursing, as evidenced by statistical texts for nursing (Knapp, 1985; Shelley, 1984; Volicer, 1984). Our anecdotal evidence about statistical curricula indicates that nonparametric statistics are given lip-service, if any service at all. Despite this lack of support, the didactic value of the Brogan approach needs to be recognized and the teaching of nonparametrics as an introduction to statistical inference considered. It goes without saying that regardless of sequence, nonparametrics should be included in master's and doctoral curricula.

Recommendations for the Integration of Statistics in Nursing Curricula

We now present a list of recommendations to guide curriculum development. As noted earlier, we refrain from proposing model curricula, mostly because many factors determine the extent to which statistics is emphasized. Also, the emphasis in this chapter on what should be expected of master's and doctoral students in terms of statistical sophistication should be a sufficient guide to the design and implementation of specific curricula.

1. The integration of statistics in nursing curricula should be guided by what is known about nursing, nursing education, nursing research, nurses, and students in nursing programs. Moreover, this comprehensive knowledge about the state of the art of the profession and discipline should be updated frequently and the curricular consequences of such updates for statistical education appraised.

2. Because of the specifics of nursing research and statistics in nursing, it is recommended that statistics courses be offered through the school of nursing, preferably by nursing faculty credentialed in (applied) statistics or

by credentialed nonnursing faculty experienced in nursing research. If this is not feasible and the teaching of statistics is to be delegated to other units within the university, content relevant to nursing should be negotiated.

3. Applied statistics should be taught and watered-down statistics avoided. Specific topics related to quantitative research in nursing should be included to the extent they are relevant to each level of education. At the doctoral level, mathematical theoretical aspects of applied statistics should be highlighted, and students should be encouraged to refine statistical techniques for nursing research. In other words, doctoral students should be given the opportunity to contribute to the area of statistics applied to nursing.

4. The rationale for teaching statistics and its relevance to inquiry in nursing should be made clear to students, in particular at those levels where research is not the primary focus (e.g., baccalaureate and master's). As Diemer (1972) showed for undergraduate dental education, the intrinsic value of a working knowledge of statistics should be highlighted if not justified if students are to be convinced of the usefulness of statistical instruction.

5. Applied multivariate statistics should be a degree requirement for doctoral education in nursing. Furthermore, it should be complemented by teaching advanced statistical topics that are intrinsic to nursing.

6. At the doctoral level in particular, it might be desirable to impose a minimum level of mathematical sophistication, or at least previous statistical coursework at the baccalaureate or master's level. Although our evidence is anecdotal, there appears to be a strong association between mathematical sophistication, introductory statistical coursework at the baccalaureate level, and Quantitative GRE-scores. Students deficient in quantitative skills but with otherwise excellent credentials for admission should be counseled accordingly. We concur with Lefkon et al. (1976) that calculus should not be a prerequisite and that applied statistics can be taught successfully to students with less mathematical sophistication.

7. Although a merely computational focus should be avoided and computer applications stressed instead, arithmetic difficulty should be considered. At the introductory level, beginning with nonparametric statistics might be beneficial (Brogan, 1980a, 1980b; see also Lefkon et al., 1976). At the intermediate and advanced level, it might be useful to teach the geometry of univariate, bivariate, and multivariate statistics before introducing actual procedures.

8. Except perhaps at the baccalaureate level, research methods and statistics should be separate but interrelated courses. Close correspondence should exist between the content of both types of courses.

9. The last recommendation applies in first instance to doctoral education, yet it may also apply to baccalaureate and master's education. The issue at stake is which segment of the student body should be targeted most. It is our recommendation that statistical instruction be offered such that the

average students are promoted and the best are stimulated, and we hope for the best for the weak. In the education of scientists there is no justification for under-stimulating the best and those with potential.

Conclusion

The chapter provided a framework for the design and implementation of statistics and quantitative science in nursing curricula. The focus was on the training of scholars and scientists, and the knowledge and skills required of them by the scientific community at large. Instead of offering prescriptive advice and model curricula, we opted for the analysis of determinants, the discussion of issues, and the formulation of contextual recommendations.

REFERENCES

Abraham, I. L. (1984). Non-statistical aspects of teaching statistics in nursing. *Bulletin on Teaching of Statistics in the Health Sciences* (American Statistical Association), Fall 1984, No. 38, 1–5.

Brogan, D. R. (1980a). A program of teaching and consultation in research methods and statistics for graduate students in nursing. *American Statistician, 34*, 26–33.

Brogan, D. R. (1980b). An integrated approach to training in research methodology and statistics. *International Journal of Nursing Studies, 17*, 101–106.

Brogan, D. R. (1982). Professional socialization to a research role: Interest in research among graduate students in nursing. *Research in Nursing and Health, 5*, 113–122.

Colton, T. (1975). An inventory of biostatistics teaching in American and Canadian medical schools. *Journal of Medical Education, 50*, 596–604.

Diemer, R. M. (1972). Teaching of statistics in dental schools. *Journal of Dental Education, 36*, 40–43.

Fitzpatrick, J. J., & Abraham, I. L. (1987). Towards the socialization of scholars and scientists. *Nurse Educator, 12*(3), 23–25.

Knapp, R. G. (1985). *Basic statistics for nurses*, 2nd ed. New York: Wiley.

Lefkon, R. G., Fletcher, M. J., & Derderian, J. C. (1976). Statistics without calculus for secondary through doctoral programs. In J. R. O'Fallon & J. Service (Eds.), *Modular instruction in statistics*. Washington, DC: American Statistical Association.

Passos, J. V., & Stallings, A. A. (1973). An introduction of concepts of measurement and statistics to sophomore nursing students. *Nursing Research, 22*, 248–253.

Shelley, S. I. (1984). *Research methods in nursing and health*. Boston: Little, Brown & Company.

Shelton, B. J. (1979). Research components in baccalaureate programs in nursing. *Journal of Nursing Education, 18*(5), 22–33.

Volicer, B. J. (1984). *Multivariate statistics for nursing research*. Orlando, FL: Grune & Stratton.

Comment

On the Prioritization of Statistical Content in Curricula

JOEL W. AGER, Ph.D.

It is unquestionably important to chart the course for curriculum development related to statistics and quantitative science programs. Equally important is the order of priorities that should be part of any curriculum development effort. The following comments are organized in two parts. In the first part, some personal biases and concerns are stated. The second part gives suggestions for assigning priorities to statistical content in nursing curricula.

Biases and Concerns

A first bias is that design, measurement, and statistical issues in nursing research do not differ much from those encountered in research in other disciplines, particularly the behavioral and health sciences. The specific content examined and theoretical frameworks used may be specific to nursing, but the methodological concerns are essentially the same. In this respect I am reminded of a consulting experience I had while still in graduate school. A biologist came to the Psychological Research

Center for some help with design and statistical analysis. At the end of our consultation he said he was surprised at my extensive knowledge of biology. I had to confess that I had never taken a course in biology, even in high school, and that, in fact, my actual knowledge of the subject was quite limited. When reduced to the appropriate X's and Y's, however, his research problem was a familiar one. I should add that the statistical consultant must always ask the right questions from the consultee to ensure that the relevant substantive aspects of the problem are understood.

Another bias is that students should have a thorough grounding in the simpler and more basic statistical techniques and their rationales before being exposed to more complex designs and statistical analyses. It is good to spend considerable time, even at the graduate level, on techniques for assessing bivariate relationships, including rank order techniques. The topics of probability, hypothesis testing, power, and confidence intervals should be thoroughly explored in this context. Only after these fundamentals are covered can the more complex analysis of variance designs and multiple regression analysis be addressed. Multivariate techniques should come only after this background has been established.

A final bias is my concern is that students may become overly dependent on the computer. It may be wise to have them do a few problems by hand, in part so that they have some contact with the raw data. Another way to facilitate familiarity with the basic data is to run univariate and bivariate frequency distributions prior to conducting the main analyses. Probably few researchers devote much effort to such preliminary analysis.

Prioritization in Statistical Curriculum Development

STUDENTS AND FACULTY

The preparation and motivation of students in advanced nursing programs for statistics and quantitative methods constitute a major problem. It would help if the empirical and research basis of nursing knowledge were given much more emphasis in the rest of the curriculum. It is important that this emphasis begin with the very first undergraduate courses. In academic programs, faculty should attempt to instill in students a scientific, skeptical, and empirical way of thinking. Research methods and statistics courses would then be seen, it is hoped, as fitting more naturally into the nursing curriculum, rather than as an isolated and onerous requirement having little to do with the rest of nursing content and practice.

With regard to staffing for a quantitative sequence at the graduate level, the most important consideration is that the people teaching at this level be qualified by training and experience. This means that, at the present time, in many doctoral programs the quantitative sequence, or parts of it, will have to be taken in other departments. As more doctorally prepared nurses also become trained as statistics and measurement specialists, it will be increasingly possible to staff the quantitative sequence within schools of nursing. The main advantage of in-house staffing, it should be noted, is not for the students but for the faculty. By teaching at the advanced level the faculty members will have a better opportunity of keeping up with current developments. Schools of nursing will also be better able to justify nursing faculty training in statistics if the quantitative teaching is done in the school.

GOALS AND APPROPRIATE LEVEL OF
A GRADUATE QUANTITATIVE METHODS SEQUENCE

While the teaching of watered-down statistics is certainly not being advocated here, it should be emphasized that a major goal of coursework should be the development of skills to select a statistical analysis appropriate for the research question being asked and the type of data. Experience dictates that this is not so easy a task, even for students with backgrounds in mathematics, mathematical statistics, and computerized data analysis. It involves identifying the independent and dependent variables and their assumed levels of measurement, along with considerations of the distributions of the variables and the assumptions of the proposed analyses. More difficult questions relate to the kinds and degrees of assumption violations that can be tolerated without jeopardizing the validity of the technique.

Another specific goal of a course sequence would be to enable students to *troubleshoot* their analyses, whether by hand or computer. That is, students should be able to recognize statistical results that are not reasonable given the data. Obvious and simple examples are means outside the range of scores, negative sums of squares or variances, and correlations greater than one in absolute value. A multiple correlation less than the highest zero order correlation is another example. Such errors in computation occur more often than one would think, even in computer analyses.

A calculus requirement is not necessary for an applied statistics sequence in nursing. Although matrix algebra is useful in the study of multivariate methods, one can go fairly extensively into the subject using the notion of linear composites of variables. The major requirements, however, are the ability to think abstractly and flexibly and to be able to apply some degree of common sense to a given analysis problem.

CONTENT AND SEQUENCE

The topics suggested in Chapter 2 for inclusion in curricula are important for nurse researchers. But one ought to ask whether it is feasible to cover most or all of these in a required quantitative sequence. Of course, this depends on the amount of time and number of courses allotted to the sequence. But *should* all topics be required? Perhaps not. A possible alternative would be to establish a basic body of content in quantitative methods to be required of all doctoral students, say, in a three-semester sequence. The more advanced topics would be covered in additional seminars targeted specifically to those students minoring in quantitative methods and any others who might be interested in advanced quantitative training. Such seminars could be given jointly with other departments and disciplines, particularly if low enrollments were a problem.

For the required sequence, one might cover in the first two courses the basic bivariate techniques, the various ANOVA and ANCOVA designs, rank order techniques, and multiple regression. The inclusion of measurement topics, including test construction, for up to one half a semester would be desirable. This is not typically done, and measurement is often a gap in students' preparation. The idea of a required multivariate course for doctoral students is a good one, and this could be the third course in the required sequence. In addition to the topics relevant to nursing research listed in the preceding chapter, one might want to cover such topics and techniques as multidimensional scaling; cluster analysis; structural models, including LISREL; logistic regression and probit analysis; Bayesian methods; jackknifing and empirical Bayesian estimation; exploratory data analysis; and techniques for handling outliers, censored data sets, and missing data. Advanced measurement topics might include generalizability theory, item response theory, and methods for assessing interrater agreement. Meta-analysis and issues in sampling might also be included. Topics for the seminars might vary some from year to year, depending on the interests of students and faculty. As it is unlikely that a single faculty member would be conversant with all or even most of these topics, team teaching and graduate student reports could be utilized for some of the presentations.

Conclusion

Abraham et al., in Chapter 2, have presented an ambitious and challenging set of goals for quantitative training in nursing. Given the complexity and characteristics of nursing research problems, the student and faculty effort that this level of training would require is entirely justified. Even the partial fulfillment of the goals outlined would represent a significant advance in graduate nursing education. In fact, the day can be envisioned when nursing research will be known for its vigor and doctorally prepared nurse researchers viewed as the quantitative experts on interdisciplinary health research teams.

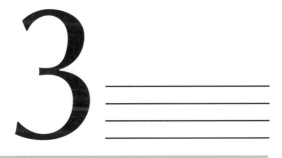

The Incipient
Paradigm Shift
in Statistical Computing

SAMUEL SCHULTZ II, Ph.D.

According to Kuhn (1962), paradigms—the collections of tools, techniques, procedures, and methods (bags of tricks)—are the primary vehicle that allows scientists to practice their craft. Paradigm shifts are the transitions from a paradigm (or set of paradigms) to a new paradigm (or set of paradigms) for a particular scientific community. Kuhn (1962) also believes that science, in fact, does not proceed in a smooth, orderly fashion but is full of quantum leaps and scientific revolutions. In his examination of the structure of scientific revolutions, Kuhn (1962) suspected that incipient paradigm shifts precede scientific revolutions.

Viewing developments in computing as incipient paradigm shifts, this chapter discusses the progress of statistical computing over the past two decades, projects changes for the future, and attempts to forecast the impact of this progress upon the producers, engineers, and practitioners of nursing knowledge. It also reviews issues that require appraisal and development by the leaders of the profession.

History

For the sake of argument, the history of statistical computing is broken into six periods, based upon the predominant mode of data management and analysis for each period. This breakdown is as follows:

Before 1965—Calculators and pencils
1965–1970—Emergence of mainframes
1970–1975—Emergence of time sharing
1975–1980—Conversational computing and database management
1980–1985—Microcomputer revolution

Each period is discussed and illustrated with examples and personal experiences.

1. *Prior to 1965*, the desktop electromechanical calculator served as the basis for statistical computing. Between 1960 and 1965 the hand calculator began to appear under the technological initiative of Texas Instruments, soon to be followed by many imitators. Calculating a simple *t*-test with 30

subjects or less on a desktop calculator was an arduous task. Performing a simple factor analysis with minimal rotation was a nearly impossible task requiring many weeks of computation.

2. In the period from *1965 to 1970* the emergence of mainframe computer technology gave scientists the ability to do simple and advanced statistical analyses in what was often described as a "flash." Yet that "flash" was in fact an interminable sequence of (new) arduous tasks with arcane languages and procedures. Often the "flash" took far more time than comparable analyses on the prevalent desktop mechanical calculators from the pre-1965 period.

This period also saw the emergence of IBM's Scientific Subroutine Package (SSP) and the UCLA's Biomedical Data (BMDP) statistical package. These developments were seen as a revolution, for they suddenly permitted the calculation of complex analyses of variance, such as the repeated measures ANOVA with missing data, analysis of covariance, and multivariate analysis of variance.

Another characteristic of this period was the move of data and calculation from the research environment to the computing center some geographical distance away. However there were very few computing facilities available to nurses in academe or service since, indeed, research as a legitimate activity for nurses was not yet widely accepted.

In 1969 we began what, to our knowledge, was one of the first (if not the first) statistical computing laboratory for nurses in an academic setting (Schultz, 1982). What was exciting at that time was to be able to sit at a 110-baud teletype machine and analyze a simple two-way mixed design analysis of variance in less than one minute from command entry to output. Operations were far from perfect, and tremendous amounts of preparation had to occur prior to the actual computing event, but there was an aura of magic surrounding the event and its products. It also beckoned the next paradigm shift for statistical computing, the revolution in remote-access and time-shared computing.

3. The years from *1970 to 1975* represented a significant change in statistical computation. During this period, because of the advent of time-sharing systems, data could be entered at a remote terminal and sent via hardware or telephone to a mainframe at some distant point. A parallel shift occurred in statistical software with the increased maturity of some more complex statistical software packages, such as SPSS and SAS, among others. Although these systems were primarily batch oriented in design, one could effect a sort of interactive analytical system by activating what was called remote batch. Just as in the earlier period one put together a stack of control cards of a "job" to be keypunched and taken across campus to the Computing Center, one could now type them in at a remote terminal, "submit" them, and get an answer rather reasonably and quickly. Later in this period, the arrival of the IBM 2741 (or Selectric Typewriter terminal) and a somewhat higher transmission speed made for better performance. However,

scientists and their staff still had to deal with arcane parameter languages for most of these statistical systems. Although these systems made researchers more oblivious to the intricacies of calculation, compensatory time was *not* spent in thinking more about the structure of the problem. It was spent on the new intricacies of the time-sharing language or statistical specification language.

What also became obvious to people during this period was the need for users to be able to set up *their own* analyses and analyze *their own* data. The need for more "user-friendly" software was recognized. Too much time was being spent on irrelevant technical details related to computing, and too little time was spent on thinking about data analysis and the structure of one's research.

Still within the period of 1970–1975 a series of programs by the University of Michigan Statistical Research Laboratory, Babystat and then Constat, attempted to deal with these problems. These programs were conversational front-end packages to a collection of statistical programs culled from the best of the BMDP, SSP, and other series. Commands were such that, with relative ease, analysis subroutines could be performed in a context that reduced preoccupation with the program itself and emphasized statistical problem solving instead. These conversational systems indeed allowed users more or less to ignore the fine structure of the computer details, and instead encouraged them to focus on their research. In 1972 the Michigan Interactive Data Analysis System (MIDAS), a statistical package developed in house at the University of Michigan, represented a major milestone in the development of such systems.

During the years 1970–1975, we also constructed a *Guide for Analyzing Data* (GAD). This guide was converted into a program that allowed researchers to reveal information about the fundamental structure of their hypotheses, data, and research and to make decisions about which statistical model(s) to select in order to answer the questions posed. Unfortunately, efforts like this were often considered "cookbook statistics" designed to lead to poor analytical procedure, because statistical advice in the form of a statistician was not present.

4. During the next period, from *1975 to 1980*, conversational statistical computing became standard methodology through the development of reliable time-sharing hardware and the appearance of mini- and microcomputer hardware. Although the most successful large-scale statistical computing packages continued to operate as batch or pseudo-batch systems, systems such as MIDAS matured into powerful, general purpose statistical utilities. Yet their power, coupled with the addition of higher-speed data transmission and CRT terminals, brought the questionable habit of ransacking databases, with total disregard for fundamental statistical issues as well as a continuing lack of regard for analysis of fundamental structure of hypotheses, data, and research questions.

Statistical computing during this period became so successful that the computer became the idiom about which all revolved. The research process may in some circumstances have suffered, as conceivably even naive neophytes could collect data, put these data into the computer, and analyze them. Whether any of the analyses were correct, whether the hypotheses were properly translated into suitable statistics, and whether legitimate results were interpreted adequately into readable English were other matters altogether. Further, the rapid emergence of other computer tools at the end of this period, such as database managers, editors and word processors, and teleconferencing, allowed a great deal more computing power but did not necessarily yield significant enhancements to the analytical log.

From an epistemological perspective, it is also important to point out that the success of statistical computing in the execution of complex analyses of variance and related models (primarily by social scientists) may have led to a predetermined methodology in nursing research constrained by the structure of analysis of variance. Although social science was well aware of the increasing emphasis on quasi-experimentation, and although nursing saw the need for methodologies attuned to research in field settings, the enthusiasm related to computing traditional experimental models may have slowed scientific developments. One could say that this most likely was a case of the statistical and technological tail wagging the professional dog.

With the emergence of the Apple II and Radio Shack microcomputers in the late 1970s, yet another revolution in computing occurred. Soon a number of computing tools operating on mainframes were becoming available on microcomputers, though initially in reduced form. It was interesting to observe how "die-hard" mainframe users attempted to ignore the potential, capability, and usefulness of microcomputer technologies.

5. Finally, the period from *1980 until 1985* was perhaps the most dramatic, not only in the history of computing but in the history of academic research and all of science. The deployment of relatively inexpensive microcomputers has brought computing back from the computing center to the research environment. A recent set of papers (Abraham & Schultz, 1986; Schultz & Abraham, 1986) reviewed the characteristics of current microcomputer technology and linked these to the many responsibilities and tasks associated with scientific activity in nursing. Obviously, the move by statistical computing from a central facility to the specific research environment poses upon schools of nursing intense demands for developing computing resources.

It should also be recognized that, in spite of the fact that statistical computing has become more accessible and that the number of tools is nearly as wide as the current theories of statistics, it is not clear that this change has in any significant way affected the scientific–analytical processes of nurse researchers. Similarly, it is not clear that the arrival of relatively inexpensive and highly available statistical computing has enhanced or will enhance the quality of the methodologies and outcomes of nursing research. This brings us back to the basic issue that making resources of any kind available does not guarantee utilization of these resources or scientific productivity. The promotion of statistical computing in nursing research is not merely a statistical matter; it also concerns nursing, nursing research, statistics, computing, and science at large.

Future

What does the next decade hold and can projections be made beyond that? Generally speaking, several rapidly developing technologies related to microcomputing will continue to foster the development of powerful, rapid, and inexpensive modes of statistical computing for nursing. A brief review of these technologies is in order.

Optical disk storage and retrieval will create the ability to store gigabyte-sized databases on virtually indestructible disk media. Essentially, there will be no physical limits to the sizes of databases. Access to any data on these databases will be immediate.

Database machines, computers optimized specifically for the storage of databases, will be placed on networks throughout universities, hospitals, and other nursing settings with scientific interests. These machines will be the servers, and database input–output devices will be used to access shared data. In concordance with this, distributed database management systems with powerful relational capabilities and conversational query languages will be ubiquitous.

It is anticipated that networks will prevail widely in any environment housing information technology. The ability to concentrate and share resources within so-called regions will become commonplace, a fact that will only enhance scientific productivity.

Laser print technology, now available and inexpensive, will permit the rapid printing of results in crisp and readable form while interspersing graphics, tables, and text. Further, the generations of microcomputers containing 32-bit and 64-bit microprocessors, allowing megabytes of real and virtual storage with fast floating-point operations, will bring unlimited computational capabilities to the desktop and emulate mainframe activity. Portable microcomputers, at a cost of a few hundred dollars each, will become more commonplace than the slide rules of the 1950s and 1960s and the hand calculators of the 1960s and 1970s. Fully conversational statistical analysis systems will be available and will contain completely integrated analytical tools that combine optimal database management with (statistical) inference. Conversational interaction between one's data and these analytical tools will be as easy as human communication.

But will this technological prowess significantly affect scientific productivity in many disciplines, including nursing? The likelihood that it will *not* is considerable, unless a "linking mechanism" is implemented. This linkage may be provided by the class of computing technology called expert systems. These programs would capture the knowledge of top statisticians, and users would be able to consult with these systems for advice on the statistical analysis of their research. Applied to nursing, the availability of statistical expert systems that are specific to nursing and health research would allow the discipline to fully embrace the utility and power of the available technology in a way that can truly effectuate a major surge in scientific productivity in nursing.

Integrating expert system technology into nursing research should be approached with the necessary caution. Indeed, what will be lost if statistical expert systems are used? Could statistics be forgotten as a science taught to graduate students? The answer may lie in whether these expert systems would have merely a statistical focus or whether they would also include matters related to quantitative methodology at large. In our opinion, one of the primary uses of expert systems in research methodology is to see that the proper questions are asked and that they are answered properly. Expert systems should not just take researchers by the hand through a deductive or inferential process leading to a solution; instead, they should be able to "question themselves" and to do work that even the sophisticated human expert may not always be able to perform satisfactorily.

Conclusion

Perhaps the most important issue to recognize in the entire matter of the integration of statistical computing into nursing research is that information is *not* knowledge. Until now, information handling has been emphasized at the expense of knowledge handling. We need to begin to move into an era of knowledge engineering for nurses. Leaders in nursing must reassess the roles that conventional mechanisms have played in the advancement and utilization of nursing knowledge. It is necessary to retain the conventional mechanisms for transferring information into knowledge, such as graduate and undergraduate curricula, grant and manuscript review, print media distribution, and utilization of textbooks as primary vehicles for distributing knowledge beyond "theory" and the "clinical experience." Yet also needed is commitment at the highest leadership level to policies that support the development of knowledge engineering based upon current and developing expert systems technology.

As Winston Churchill said, "I pass with relief from the tossing sea of cause and theory to the firm ground of result and fact." We submit to you that expert systems technology applied to statistics and quantitative methods will allow us to pass with relief from the tossing sea of information to the firm ground of knowledge in and about nursing.

REFERENCES

Abraham, I. L., & Schultz, S. (1986). Interfacing microcomputers and nursing research—I. Management and analysis of research data. *Western Journal of Nursing Research, 8*, 386–391.

Kuhn, T. S. (1962). *The structure of scientific revolutions*. Chicago: University of Chicago Press.

Schultz, S. (1982). A model computing laboratory for university schools of nursing: The Michigan experience. In *Proceedings of the Sixth Annual Symposium on Computer Applications in Medical Care*. Los Angeles: IEEE Computer Society.

Schultz, S., & Abraham, I. L. (1986). Interfacing microcomputers and nursing research—II. Dissemination of research findings and project management. *Western Journal of Nursing Research, 8*, 473–477.

Comment

On Statistical Expert Systems

LEE-HWA JANE, M.S.N., R.N.

As stated in Chapter 3, there are many changes in statistical computing affecting scientific activity in nursing. Among them, statistical expert systems are perhaps the most promising technology that will be seen in the near future. It is important to clarify what expert systems are and how they may confirm the expectations that are currently being placed upon them by the statistical community and by scientific communities at large.

Expert Systems

As an introduction and for matters of clarification, two definitions of expert system are presented. According to Feigenbaum (cited in Harmon & King, 1985), an expert system is "an intelligent computer program that uses knowledge and interface procedures to solve problems that are difficult enough to require significant human expertise for their solution" (p. 5). Hahn (1985) defined expert systems as information technology in which "the knowledge of an expert is built into a computer program, enabling it to emulate the process that the expert follows in attacking a problem" (p. 1).

Expert systems have been applied in various fields. To cite a

TABLE 1. Steps in Data Analysis As Performed by
Human Statistical Experts

Step	Tasks
1. Problem–solution definition	Definition of the statistical problem Screening of the data Selection of the appropriate models for solution
2. Data analysis	Statistical inference
3. Interpretation	Explanation of the results obtained through statistical inference
4. Evaluation	Pointing out of patterns and peculiarities in data Planning of further analyses

few examples, physicians use them to diagnose diseases; geologists, to locate mineral deposits; executives, to assist with complex managerial tasks; computer engineers, to configure complex computer hardware; mechanics, to aid in troubleshooting locomotive problems (Hahn, 1985; Harmon & King, 1985). Expert systems in nursing are now mostly related to clinical decision making and education (Ryan, 1985; Ozbolt, Schultz, Swain, & Abraham, 1985). In recent years, statisticians have come to realize the potential of expert systems in statistical problem solving and have initiated the development of such systems.

Statistical Expert Systems

Statistical expert systems perform tasks in a manner analogous to that of the human statistical expert. The process of statistical problem solving by humans can be broken down into four steps, as illustrated in Table 1. Step 1 is *Problem–Solution Definition*, in which the statistical problem is defined, the data are screened, and the appropriate models and methods for analyzing the data are selected. This is followed by *Data Analysis* (Step 2) and *Interpretation* (Step 3). In the final step, *Evaluation*, the patterns and peculiarities in the data are considered and further analyses may be initiated.

Ideally, a powerful statistical expert system should be able to assist users in all four steps of data analysis. As such, they would guide the user in defining the problem, developing appropriate models, selecting analytic methods, interpreting results, and planning further analyses. This kind of expert system is not yet commercially available. However, two "less intelligent" types of expert systems have been developed.

The first type is characterized by expert guidance embedded in a statistical program. This type of expert system provides assistance in the second, third, and fourth steps of data analysis; that is, in selecting data analytic strategies, interpreting the results, and considering further analyses. The second type is characterized by the ability to define problems and their solutions. This type aids users in the first step of data analysis and thus identifies analyses appropriate for the data at hand. It may also provide an explanation of its decisions when requested by the user.

Conclusion

Statistical computing indeed is now much more accessible than before. Access to a personal computer with statistical software allows almost anyone to perform statistical analyses. However, there is a danger inherent in their accessibility, in that, conceivably, people with minimal statistical sophistication may engage in statistical analysis without guidance and, therefore, with a high probability of error and inaccuracy. To avoid the danger of unguided analysis by novices and experts alike, the development of statistical expert systems that interface with statistical programs should be promoted.

REFERENCES

Hahn, G. J. (1985). More intelligent statistical software and statistical expert systems: Future directions. *The American Statistician, 39*, 1–8.

Harmon, P., & King, D. (1985). *Artificial intelligence in business*. New York: Wiley.

Ozbolt, J. G., Schultz, S., Swain, M. A. P., & Abraham, I. L. (1985). A proposed expert system for nursing practice. *Journal of Medical Systems, 9*, 57–68.

Ryan, S. A. (1985). An expert system for nursing practice: Clinical decision support. *Computers in Nursing, 4*, 77–84.

Resources and Structures to Promote Research in Nursing

JOANNE SABOL STEVENSON, Ph.D., F.A.A.N.

This chapter incorporates two complementary schemata to cover the topic. First, we go through a brief historical overview of the resources and structures developed for nursing research over the past several years in many areas of the United States. A more comprehensive discussion appears elsewhere (Stevenson, 1987). Second, we present a systems approach to go from the needs of the individual researcher to the requirements for larger system resources and structures. This segment moves from the single organization to the regional, national, and international levels.

Historical Overview of Research Development

The first center for research in the field of nursing was developed by R. Louise McManus at Teachers College, Columbia University, in 1953 (Vreeland, 1964). It was called the Institute of Research and Service in Nursing Education, and its purpose was to promote and implement research in nursing education. The first formalized nursing research center was developed at Wayne State University in 1969. Dr. Harriet Werley was recruited to be its first director. She had come to Wayne State after retirement from the military. During her preretirement years she developed a nursing research unit within the Research Institute at Walter Reed Army Hospital (Werley, 1962). This effort spawned the early clinical nursing research on care issues by Phyllis Verhonick (decubitus ulcers) and Marian Ginsberg (mouth care of patients with uremic frost), and introduced the use of small laboratory animals (rats and guinea pigs) in nursing research. In the Wayne State University effort, Werley used her previous experiences at Walter Reed but expanded her sights considerably by visiting several researchers and research centers in other disciplines and in other geographic areas. (The development of the Wayne Center was reported in *Nursing Research*, Vol. 22, No. 3, 1973 [Werley and Shea, 1973].) The purposes were to promote scientific investigations relevant to health and nursing, transmission of knowledge, utilization, research training, and interdisciplinary collaboration. A few years later the center was renamed the Center for Health Research.

The second Center for Nursing Research was developed at Ohio State University in 1972. Its purpose was to promote and facilitate nursing research—both basic research and clinical studies on care issues of concern to the discipline of nursing. The catchment area for this facilitation effort was defined geographically as the entire mid-Ohio area, and the target population included all potential nurse researchers in the area, including faculty, students, alumni, and nurses in the health care agencies and schools of nursing in the region. Research included many topics, but the major foci were women's health, family and community health, and health promotion.

Additional nursing research centers developed over the next several years. Some of these were at the University of Minnesota, the University of Nebraska, the Center for Nursing Research and Evaluation at the University of Wisconsin, Milwaukee, and others. Those research-oriented schools that did not develop centers almost without exception established some structure to develop and facilitate research. In most instances, the efforts were led by an associate or assistant dean or a director and the administrative structure was an office for research with commonalities in the staffing patterns.

Federal Funding for Nursing Research

These development efforts in the schools were significantly helped by federal funding. The first actual research grant given by the Division of Nursing, which was originally housed in the National Institute of General Medical Science, was awarded in 1955. The thirtieth anniversary of the beginning of direct federal funding of nursing research, 1985, was also the landmark legislation to move nursing research back to the National Institutes of Health (NIH).

The model of support for nursing research developed and used over a period of 30 years by the Division of Nursing is an excellent one and worth emulating on a smaller scale by institutions and organizations interested in facilitating the development of nursing research. In the beginning a high percentage of the resources was committed to researcher development. In the early days, funding priority went to the mid-career development of faculty already on the staffs in schools of nursing. Faculty Research Development Grants provided methods and statistics training and enhanced other competencies of faculty. Later, money was directed toward helping these people and some second-generation people do start-up studies, do pilot work, and seek independent funding. Still later, money was channeled primarily into predoctoral fellowships and institutional grants for the predoctoral training of nurse scientists. Most recently, postdoctoral fellowships are being stressed and given more monetary support. A group of advisors to the Division of Nursing in 1984 suggested that there be a 50–50 split of money for pre- and postdoctoral fellowships. Between 1984 and 1986, the Division of Nursing for the first time awarded institutional grants for the training of pre- and postdoctoral fellows under the direction of highly qualified research mentors.

In 1986, the National Center for Nursing Research (NCNR) within the National Institute of Health became the responsible funding agency for nursing research. During its early years, the NCNR has added several new funding mechanisms. The new grant mechanisms include the Academic Research Enhancement Award (AREA), the First Independent Research Support and Transition Award (FIRST), the Method to Extend Research in Time (MERIT), the Academic Investigator Award (AIA), the Clinical Investigator Award (CIA), the National Research Service Award (NRSA) Senior Fellowship, and the Small Business Innovation Research Award (SBIRA). These award programs have significantly boosted the research activity and research career development of the nursing community.

Resources and Structures in a Single Organization

In our final report on the Ohio State Research Development Program (Stevenson, 1975) we wrote that the three key ingredients to a successful research program are (1) talented, knowledgeable, and committed people; (2) equipment; and (3) resources and services to support the efforts of the talented, knowledgeable, and committed people and their equipment. Schlotfeldt (1973), in the final report on the Case Western Reserve University Faculty Research Development Grant, said, "development of research in any discipline must await the availability of a critical mass of prepared investigators ... and their sustained pursuit of ... knowledge are enhanced by encouragement, time, equipment, supplies, and space" (Schlotfeldt, 1973, p. 1). With those words, Schlotfeldt (1973) outlined the major needs for resources.

Batey (1978) evaluated the 12 research development programs funded by the Division of Nursing during the late 1960s and early 1970s. Schools that used the grants most successfully for continuing research productivity had several characteristics, of which the most relevant were: research as a visible, accountable, and formal part of the table of organization; an administrative policy that reflects research as an expected goal of the school; the use by a school of its own funds to seed research; a formal reward system for promotions and tenure that includes research productivity; and faculty who accept the triad of teaching, research, and service as professional responsibilities.

Tables 4-1 and 4-2 are comprehensive matrices of resources, services,

TABLE 4–1. RESOURCES FOR NURSING RESEARCH

Facilities	Staffing	Services	Equipment	Incentives	Activities	Funding	
						Intramural	Extramural
Wet/dry labs., research offices, secretarial space, data storage–equipment space, team meeting area, library/reading room	Administrator–Facilitator, cadre scholars–researchers, data processors, fiscal personnel, programmer(s)–computer specialists, research assts.–associates, consultants	Typing–word processing, library search, messenger, fiscal–purchasing, consultation (e.g., content, methods), travel funds	Secretarial, storage, data collection–data processing, computation, data files	Promotion–tenure, recruitment, contracts, pilot money, internal funding competition, 9-mo. contracts, sabbaticals–leaves, mid-career retraining	Research committee, seminars–brown bag, group consultation, individ. consult., informal presentation–conf., symposia, lecture series, visiting prof. series, newsletters	Hard money, dvlpmt. funds, competitive intramural grants, overhead recovery, small grants, travel grants, sabbaticals, mini-international programs	Local–Reg'l–nat'l foundations, voluntary assoc., ANF, Sigma Theta Tau Int'l., NAACOG, AACN, federal state, and local gov't, int'l sources

TABLE 4–2. STRUCTURES FOR NURSING RESEARCH

Administrative Structures	Research–Scholar Structures	Centralized Structure for Research	Boundary Crossing for Research	Larger Social Structures, I: Reg–Natl. & Int'l	Larger Social Structures, II: Prof. Nsg. Organizations	Structures for Monetary Support	Larger Social System Influence and Infiltration
Supportive central admin., supportive dean–nursing director, mission & milieu of parent institution, adequacy of all funding, research oversight–evaluation board; entity for research development	Critical mass, complementary areas of expertise, conducive table of organization (e.g., academic or clinical depts.), spirit of cooperation & collaboration, brownian movement, peer support system	Team or group, office, center, institute, other	Org. set-up of parent organization, milieu of parent organization, interdepartmental cooperation–collaboration, multidisciplinary milieu, cross-discipline partnerships, researcher–clinician partnerships	Research societies, networking structures, interest groups/ sections, multi-organization structures, consortia	ANA (cabinet–council), AAN, AACN, NLN, regional societies, specialty organizations, ICN, other	Local–reg–natl. foundations, ANF, Sigma Theta Tau Int'l; federal, state, and local Govt.; pre- & post-doc. fellowships; research career awards; new invest. awards; mid-career awards; sr. scholar awards; instit. awards	Inform public—media/consumers, review group membership, placement on funding agency boards, influence Congress & foundation boards, influence policy and priorities of HHS–other funding agencies

and structures that were found in a survey of literature and nursing organizations.

Table 4-1 focuses on resources. The major topic headings are facilities, support staff, services, equipment, incentives–pressures, formalized development activities, and funding sources. Under facilities, for example, there is a listing of the kinds of research facilities found around the country. Not every organzation has them all, but each does exist somewhere. Staffing is self-explanatory and so are many of the other categories. Funding resources are broken down into sources within the institution (e.g., university) and from without (e.g., federal government).

Table 4-2 shows the structures for research that exist around the country. The categories here are administrative structures, researcher–scholar structures, the housing of the research facilitation effort, the structures for boundary crossing, larger social structures, and structures in the environment (local to international) for monetary support.

Conclusion

Resources and structures to support nursing research are necessary at many system levels: the individual level of the single nurse researcher through the single organizational entity that employs that nurse and through the parent organization of the entity. The employing organization, through its leadership, is the most important link in the chain of nursing research development. This organization, through its administrators, recruits research-competent people, initiates and supports the development of organizational structures, and provides adequate staff and material to help the researchers do the work of science (Stevenson, 1979). Beyond the grassroots level, nursing organizations, societies, policy-making groups, and lobbying groups are extremely important for the long-term viability of resources and structures for nursing research.

Nurse researchers play an important role in keeping our needs and the products of our research in the public eye. A first step is to inform the consumer public, lawmakers, and policymakers about nursing research—what it is, what it produces, how its outcomes are useful, what happens to its outcomes, who can do it, where it can be done, and what resources are required to do it.

Second, our several publics must hear about the products of nursing research almost as a daily routine—bombarded with the concept and the outcomes of nursing research over and over again—in testimony, in local and national newspapers and popular magazines of health articles, on talk shows, in documentaries, and so on. The public image of nursing must come to include nursing science.

Third, nurses must get appointed or elected to more boards, councils, committees of funding agencies, private foundations, voluntary organizations, and governmental bodies. This infiltration by nurses is critical to the policy-making and monetary allocation decisions of these bodies. So the more respected and assertive nurses we can get strategically placed, the more influence nursing can have on policy decisions, which in turn affect the allocation of resources and development of structures for nursing research in the larger sociopolitical arena.

REFERENCES

Batey, M. V. (1978). *Research development in university schools of nursing* (Publication No. HRA 78–67). Hyattsville, MD: U.S. Department of Health, Education, and Welfare.

Brand, K. P., & Martinson, I. M. (1976). Evolution of a nursing research center. *Nursing Outlook, 24,* 704–707.

Schlotfeldt, R. M. (1973). *Creating a climate for nursing research.* Cleveland: Frances Payne Bolton School of Nursing, Case Western Reserve University.

Stevenson, J. S. (1975). *Research development program in nursing.* Columbus: Ohio State University Research Foundation.

Stevenson, J. S. (1979). Support for an emerging social institution. In F. S. Downs & J. W. Fleming (Eds.), *Issues in nursing research.* Norwalk, CT: Appleton-Century-Crofts.

Stevenson, J. S. (1987). Forging a research discipline. *Nursing Research, 36,* 60–64.

Vreeland, E. M. (1964). Nursing research programs of the public health service. *Nursing Research, 13,* 148–158.

Werley, H. H. (1962). Promoting the research dimension in the practice of nursing through the establishment and development of a Department of Nursing in an institute of research. *Military Medicine, 127,* 219–231.

Werley, H. H., & Shea, F. P. (1973). The first center for research in nursing: Its development, accomplishments, and problems. *Nursing Research, 22,* 217–231.

Comment

Linking the Scientist to Research Resources and Structures

W. RICHARD COWLING III, Ph.D., R.N.

The previous chapter provides an overview of the historical record of resources and structures for nursing research in the United States. In addition, it presents a systems approach to needs of the individual researcher through requirements for larger system resources and structures. The comments offered here are elaborations on some of the issues identified in Chapter 4.

The employing agency was identified as the most important link in the chain of nursing research development with the agency's leadership emphasized as the major factor. Leadership for promoting nursing research in the academic institution as well as the service setting has been given little attention in the nursing research literature. Although some schools of nursing have begun to implement programs of study aimed at developing the nurse executive–administrator for academic or service settings as part of a larger Ph.D. curriculum, little attention has been given to the development of the researcher as a leader for promoting scientific inquiry at various systems levels. In addition, the distinctive features of the role of the administrator in research programs at the institutional level have not been studied and approached systematically to extend current knowledge about research administration to the degree that is needed. Elements of research structures presented in the matrices in the preceding chapter could serve as a guide to developing education program content for preparing nursing research administrators. These matrices could also serve as general content for anyone to understand and analyze the role of the researcher in a larger organizational context.

It is essential to give attention to the individual nurse researcher in an organization. For structures to be effective, they must provide the means through which resources of that particular structure reach the individual researcher and promote sustained scientific productivity. One of the critical issues in structuring research environments is how the structure can accommodate the perceived needs of an individual researcher while also considering the total research program of the organization. Structuring research environments and programs to facilitate the linkages between individual researchers might address this issue, but a strong sense of shared governance of research programming seems essential to the motivation of most individual researchers. Specific mechanisms, such as faculty involvement in research committees that make decisions about resources or in advisory capacities for educational programs, heighten this sense of shared governance in research administration. Structuring should also provide mechanisms for rewarding and recognizing the accomplishments of individual researchers, such as through publication of achievements in school and university newsletters. Increasing consideration of individual recognition and reward could increase productivity. Finally, the structure of research must give attention to the career development of the individual researcher in the context of the total program of research. This requires research administrators to be continually conscious of how the individual researcher's own program of research may fit with the goals of the particular research organization, from the time of recruitment of the researcher onward. Consideration should also be given to providing research career counseling for new Ph.D. graduates and for researchers making a change in area of focus.

Beyond productivity, creativity and innovation as well as enhanced quality in scientific endeavors of the core researchers need to be given consideration in evaluating the resource richness and structuring of research programs. Too frequently the major indicator of success of a research program is limited to productivity alone. One of the major challenges of research managers and administrators may well be to make significant contributions to program evaluation applied to the research program and research environment. Emphasis on the potential indicators of quality and creativity in research programs is needed. At the same time, variables that affect quality and creativity in research programs need to be identified and studied.

Moving from the individual researcher to the organization that employs researchers, it is likely that collaboration or unification models for nursing education and service will have a significant impact on structures and resources for research. Clear delineation of education–service relationships with regard to the research goals of both is crucial to the success of programmatic efforts. The allocation of resources will be dependent to a large degree on the structure of both service and education programs for research, that is, whether there is a joint structure of independent structures with some sharing and collaboration. The potential for enhancement of scientific endeavors in both number and quality is great, but it is clear that the interests and values of clinicians and researchers need to be equally represented for this enhancement to occur.

Another important area that deserves attention as a structure and resource problem in nursing research is that of the needs of the beginning researcher. It is evident that the development of research proposals and submission for funding requires resources that go beyond those often available to the beginning researcher. The amount of time spent to generate a literature review in many research areas alone is significant. Resources such as research assistants are usually allocated to those who have obtained the necessary funding. Again, structure plays a central role in providing mechanisms for allocating resources for the development of research, particularly for the beginning researcher, as well as for the implementation of research. Ways to track the investment of resources for research development from the generation of ideas to the formalization of research proposals, and the returns on such investments, are needed to provide the impetus for greater resource allocation at the originating points. Research administrators would be wise to consider the investment potential of providing increasing resources for research development and seek innovative ways to fund this significant phase of the research process.

Lastly, it is important to attend to the public image of nursing as a science and the role of nurses on boards, councils, and committees that influence policy and allocation of funds for nursing research. The public image of nursing as a science can best be strengthened by bringing much of what we do as scientists to the attention of media sources. But we also need to give greater attention to the areas in which we can contribute as scientists. Linking our knowledge and abilities as nurse scientists to the health problems of society through systematic, directed, and programmatic efforts could contribute greatly to the image of nursing as a science. Recognition of scientific contributions through media attention will also help those elected or appointed to councils, committees, and boards realize the importance of nurses' involvement in such groups.

PART 2

Quantitative Science in Nursing Research

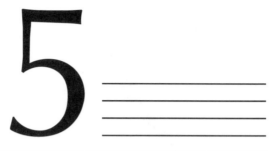

Statistics and Quantitative Methods in Medical–Surgical Nursing

BEVERLY L. ROBERTS, Ph.D., R.N.

Research is the systematic process to generate and evaluate knowledge in order to develop theories describing the interrelationships between concepts and in order to evaluate their congruency with empirical findings (Reynolds, 1971). Quantitative methods and statistics are means by which these aims are achieved. Published results of research provide the opportunity to evaluate not only the knowledge generated, but also the scientific methods used. Considering the (often two-year) period from completion of a study to its publication, the current application of statistical and quantitative methods is not reflected yet in today's publications. Insight into the current trends in applications is therefore not possible; however, published findings in a given, recent time period provide an opportunity to identify and analyze the most recent statistics and quantitative methods used. Consequently, the analysis of the application of statistics and quantitative methods used in medical–surgical nursing research, presented in this chapter, is based on articles published in *Research in Nursing and Health* and *Nursing Research* for the two-year period of June 1983 to June 1985. Although not an exhaustive sample of all research reports in the area of medical-surgical nursing, it will be apparent that the emerging trends and issues are representative of those within medical-surgical nursing at large.

Quantitative Methodologies

Investigators used experimental and quasi-experimental designs most frequently. Considering nursing's clinical component and focus on developing prescriptive theory (Dickoff & James, 1968), it is not surprising that few investigators utilized descriptive and exploratory methodologies. LeSage (1984) and Mishel (1984) were the only investigators to utilize these non-experimental methods to describe the relationships among phenomena; other investigators also isolated factors that predicted phenomena of interest (DuCette & Keane, 1984; Hubbard, Muhlenkamp, & Brown, 1984). Since the extent of existing knowledge about these phenomena was limited, descriptive and exploratory methodologies were appropriate.

Several investigators used ex post facto designs to examine the effects of a preexisting independent variable. For example, Murphy (1984) examined the effects of loss of a loved one or loss of residence due to a natural disaster on stress and health of individuals. Attempting to identify differences between those persons who suffered a loss of a loved one, those who suffered a loss of a residence, and those who had no losses, she noted the weakness of this design, because no predisaster measurements were available. Thus, the design limited the causal inferences that could be made. Penckoffer and Holm (1984) and O'Connor (1983) studied persons who recently underwent coronary artery bypass surgery. These investigators attempted to strengthen the ex post facto design by obtaining pretest measurements of recalled information. These questionable pretest measurements and the absence of a comparison group, however, prevented true causal inferences about the effects of bypass surgery.

When existing knowledge indicated possible intervention strategies, investigators attempted to utilize experimental designs. Yet few investigators used randomization in the selection or assignment of subjects, because of the small numbers of persons meeting the criteria for selection and the difficult or limited access to populations of interest. Consequently, quasi-experimental designs were often used instead.

Two issues arise with quasi-experimental designs: the ability to make causal inferences and the equivalency of subgroups of subjects. As to the first issue, no studies were identified in which the research design did not allow causal inference. However, it is probably the second issue that is most pertinent. Equivalency of groups occurs when the effects of confounding variables are controlled by randomization. In contrast, nonrandom samples may vary with respect not only to the variable of interest, but also to other variables related to these variables (Levy & Lemeshow, 1983). Before control of these variables is possible, significant differences between the groups must be identified. This is accomplished by statistical analyses that compare the groups on the variables of interest and other variables considered to be related to them. Investigators used a variety of statistical techniques, but those most often used were the t-test and the F-test.

Where the groups were not equivalent and the significant covariate was not controlled, analysis of covariance (ANCOVA) and blocking were the most common techniques for controlling confounding in between-group differences. Bohachick (1984) and Harris and Hyman (1984) used pretest measurements as covariates to adjust for initial differences in the groups; Sexton and Munro (1985) used ANCOVA to control for the effects of age and occupation on the variables of interest in their study. The second technique, blocking according to the quantity of a confounding variable, characterized studies in which control of the presumed effects of anxiety on dependent variables was necessary (Scott, Oberst, & Bookbinder, 1984; Sime

& Libera, 1985). In these studies, initial measurements of anxiety were used to place subjects in homogeneous groups according to level of anxiety. The variation related to the effects of this blocking variable could then be isolated from the variation associated with error. The advantage of blocking is the fewer assumptions needed to be met than in ANCOVA. Interestingly, none of the investigators who used ANCOVA reported testing for the statistical assumptions governing this approach.

Regardless of whether experimental or quasi-experimental methodologies were used, most investigators utilized one-way or factorial analysis of variance (ANOVA) designs to determine treatment effects and to make comparisons between groups. However, a trend toward more complex and sophisticated designs that permit the detection of the potential effects of other factors (treatments, order of treatments, and interactions) was noted. In particular, repeated measures and mixed designs were often used. These designs pose less sample size demand to obtain the same amount of information. Further, they allow isolation of within-subject variability and are associated with greater precision and power (Cohen & Cohen, 1975; Pedhazur, 1982).

Latin-squares is another complex design that not only reduces the number of subjects required for the effects examined, but also allows for determination of differences associated with the order in which various treatments are introduced (Hays, 1978; Kirk, 1968). This design was used in a study of cardiovascular response to talking (Thomas, Friedmann, Lottes, Gresty, Miller, & Lynch, 1984). With a smaller number of subjects, these designs provide more power and information about effects and their interactions than simpler designs. Considering the difficulty in accessing, recruiting, and retaining subjects in clinical research, these complex designs should be used more often.

Information About Phenomena and Effects

Information about phenomena and experimental effects was frequently lost by rescaling measurements from interval or ratio levels to ordinal level (Diekman, 1984; Vanbree, Hollerbach, & Brooks, 1984; Wells & Giden, 1984). This rescaling to a lower level was associated with a loss of information about the phenomena. In addition, less powerful nonparametric statistics were then required for analysis of these rescaled measurements. Wells and Giden (1984) offered no explanation for rescaling measurements, and Diekman (1984) defended it on the basis of the small sample size of the study. Vanbree et al. (1984) justified the rescaling by noting that repeated measurements are not independent and that, therefore, the assumption to use parametric tests was violated. This, in fact, is an invalid justification: the analysis of variance for repeated measures incorporates the fact that measurements must not to be independent and considers this in the analysis (Hays, 1978; Kirk, 1968). We also noted that a few investigators inappropriately selected parametric tests when the assumption of continuous levels of measurements was not met (Penckoffer & Holm, 1984; Ziemer, 1983). Spurious results may have ensued.

The most frequent error in the selection of statistical techniques was found to occur when multiple comparisons between groups were required or repeated measurements of subjects were used. Several investigators expected specific differences between groups (Fehring, 1983; Levesque, Grenier, Kerovac, & Reidy, 1984; Winslow, Lane, & Gaffney, 1985). Instead of using the more powerful planned comparisons with contrast coding specific for these differences, they used the less powerful post hoc comparisons and decreased the probability of detecting existing differences in the treatments compared (Hays, 1978). Still others used multiple t-tests without compensating for the inflation of alpha associated with these multiple tests (Rice & Johnson, 1984; Ziemer, 1983). Except for noting the differences in the means and standard deviations of the variables in each group, Dixon (1984) did not examine differences between the control group and four treatment groups that were expected by the hypotheses.

Post hoc comparisons assume that the measurements being compared are independent (Kirk, 1968). Even though repeated measures on the same subject are not independent, Winer (1971) recommended the use of post hoc comparisons to identify differences between these measurements. Winslow et al. (1985) appropriately used post hoc comparisons to examine differences in repeated cardiovascular measurements during different types of bathing. Martyn, Hansen, and Jen (1984) used these comparisons in a study of caloric intake and gastric motility in rhesus monkeys. Yet several investigators (Dressler, Smejkal, & Ruffolo, 1983; Parsons & Wilson, 1984) failed to consider post hoc comparisons of repeated measurements. Kirchoff, Rebenson-Piano, and Patel (1984) (correctly) justified not using these comparisons on the basis that repeated measurements are not independent and multiple comparisons assume independence. Those who failed to use post hoc multiple comparisons lost information about where differences in response occurred and about trends over time.

When significant interactions occur in analysis of variance, simple effects can be used to gain information about how all effects vary across a level of another effect (Pedhazur, 1982). Most analysis of variance designs used were simple one-way designs, and only two studies had results where significant interactions occurred. Sime and Libera (1985) appropriately utilized simple effects to test for the factors in the interaction, and Dixon (1984) noted the interaction but failed to examine these effects. If more complex designs are used in the future, the number of studies with significant interactions will increase.

In the future, the use of multiple correlated dependent variables may increase as well. Univariate statistical techniques do not consider the inter-correlations between these variables, and information on how these vary together as a whole is lost. Multivariate statistical techniques consider covariations among variables and integrate this information in the analyses (Green, 1978). Interpretation of multivariate analyses is more complex and difficult because of the lack of independence in the outcome variables, but these techniques provide useful information about complexly related variables. Multivariate techniques consider the complexity of the whole, whereas univariate techniques isolate the parts of the whole. Considering the variables as correlated may lead to inferences that are different from those that are reached when variables are treated independently (Rao, 1966). Investigators in only two studies used multivariate techniques (Kirchoff et al., 1984; Sime & Libera, 1985), even though there were several studies where the dependent variables were correlated and multivariate analyses would have been appropriate (Murphy, 1984; Parsons & Wilson, 1984; Sitzman, Kamuja, & Johnston, 1983; Ventura, Young, Feldman, Pastore, Pikula, & Yates, 1984; Wells & Giden, 1984).

Psychometric Studies

Seven articles included description of the results of psychometric analysis. Each instrument was linked to a theoretical construct, but investigators in only one of the studies had a theoretical basis for the number and content of the underlying dimensions of the construct (Given, Given, Gallin, & Condon, 1983). Validity and reliability were evaluated in these studies. The deficiency in these studies was the inadequate sample size for factor analysis that was used to establish construct validity.

Although no absolute rules exist and quantitative approaches are less common than rules of thumb, Kerlinger (1973) stated that the minimal sample size for factor analysis is 10 subjects for each item in the instrument. A small sample size reduces the stability of the factor structures. The samples of only two studies met this criteria (Cox, 1985; Padilla, Presant, Grant, Metter, Lipsett, & Heide, 1983). Even though they used an inadequate sample, Dawson, Schirmer, and Beck (1984) noted the instability in factor structures and assessed this by utilizing two other samples for cross-validation.

Descriptions of factor-analytic procedures were complete in most studies (Cox, 1985; Dawson et al., 1983). These descriptions included the factor-analytic procedures used and the criteria applied in the selection of factors and items comprising them. These investigators selected factors and items based not only on statistical results, but also on the conceptual meaningfulness and interpretability of these factors. Except for Cox (1985), information regarding the correlation between factors and the interpretation of this correlation was lacking.

Other techniques were used to establish validity. Several investigators had the items of the questionnaires evaluated by a panel of judges for content validity (Derdiarian & Forsythe, 1983; Jalowiec, Murphy, & Powers, 1984). Concurrent validity was established by correlations of the score on the instrument with another measure of the same construct (Dawson et al., 1984; Padilla et al., 1983). In addition, investigators used analysis of variance to determine whether groups that would be expected to differ on the construct did indeed differ. Validity of the instruments was enhanced by the utilization of these various techniques.

All investigators used Cronbach's alpha to establish the internal consistency of the whole instrument to the total score and the internal consistency of each factor isolated by factor analysis (Cox, 1985; Dawson et al., 1984; Derdiarian & Forsythe, 1983; Given et al., 1983; Jalowiec et al., 1984; Padilla et al., 1983). This information about reliability of subscales is necessary if they are to be used in future studies.

Theory Building

Theories that provide an understanding of the relationships between variables can be developed and evaluated by the statistical techniques of causal modeling and meta-analysis. Mishel (1984) was the only investigator whose purpose of study was to evaluate a theoretical model of uncertainty and stress in illness. The model testing was flawed for it consisted of attempting to reconstruct the model using correlations between the variables and multiple regressions to predict endogenous variables. This mode of constructing and evaluating a model is based not on theory, but solely on data. Correlation-based techniques such as the ones used by Mishel (1984) ignore the fact that measures of association between variables do not reflect the theoretical underpinnings of a model (Cook & Campbell, 1979). Since correlations without a theoretical model cannot be decomposed into direct, indirect, and spurious effects, they cannot be used to develop a theoretical model (Pedhazur, 1982). Development of a model must be grounded in theory, not derived from sample-specific data (Cook & Campbell, 1979; Pedhazur, 1982). Further, after reconstructing the model, Mishel (1984) used path analysis to determine and test the significance of the path coefficients. Yet causal modeling is a technique to evaluate the congruency of fit of the empirical data to the model, to determine strength of the causal linkages described by the model, and to identify the magnitude of direct, indirect, and spurious effects. It is not to be used solely for the purpose of computing path coefficients (Pedhazur, 1982).

Another technique used in theory building is meta-analysis. In this aggregate of techniques; the results of several studies of the same phenomena are examined. They quantify the level of significance of the relationship or experimental intervention and the size of the effect noted and also identify moderators of the findings (Glass, McGaw, & Smith, 1981). This technique was used in one study examining the relationship between psychoeducational interventions and length of hospital stay in 49 studies (Devine & Cook, 1983). These researchers were able to determine the changes in effect sizes found in the studies over time and to identify variables and conditions that may account for these differences. These results added support for the effect of psychoeducational interventions on hospitalization and suggested possible moderation variables.

Implications for the Future

The preponderance of experimental and quasi-experimental methodologies reflects an emphasis on determining the effects of interventions that have ready application to clinical practice. This emphasis is consistent with the ultimate goal of prescriptive theories applicable to clinical practice (Dickoff & James, 1968) and the aim of a professional discipline toward practical application of knowledge (Donaldson & Crowley, 1978).

Results of descriptive and exploratory studies are not necessarily readily applicable to the clinical setting, but they provide the basis for understanding the phenomena, developing theories, and identifying interventions. Expansion of knowledge relevant to medical-surgical nursing requires identifying relevant phenomena and selecting the methodology for research that is consistent with existing knowledge.

Since the majority of studies included in our review were clinical and required the participation of subjects who may have been difficult to recruit and retain, methodologies and designs needed to be attuned to the realities of clinical environments and clinical research. Advanced statistical methods that maximize the relevance of research under those conditions should be applied. Helpful designs include latin-squares and repeated measures. Repeated measures designs also allow for determining change over time and a description of this change. Time series and profile analysis are techniques that can be used to describe temporal changes in greater detail.

Further expansion of knowledge will also require valid and reliable instruments to operationalize concepts. Currently, investigators are utilizing appropriate techniques to evaluate the psychometric properties of instruments. As more investigators focus on concepts and phenomena about which little is known and because instruments for their measurements do not exist, more psychometric studies will be required.

Generally, investigators utilized appropriate statistical techniques for the nature of the measurements and research questions. These techniques were most frequently univariate, even though the complexity of inter-relationships between phenomena of interest to the nursing discipline has been acknowledged (Munhall, 1981). However, statistical techniques exist that are consistent with this perspective of holism, in which the whole is defined as more than the sum of its parts. Multivariate techniques consider the complexity of these interrelationships between phenomena and should be used more extensively in nursing research. Even though interpretation of the findings is more difficult than in univariate inference, multivariate techniques more adequately provide an understanding of the complex nature of the phenomena.

The systematic and objective techniques used in research focus not only on describing phenomena but also on the development and evaluation of theories. Experimental and quasi-experimental studies and mechanisms enable scientists to establish causal relationships, but causal modeling and meta-analysis are other statistical techniques that can be used to develop and evaluate theories. Considering the preponderance of studies focusing on specific interventions, these statistical techniques can be utilized to move beyond empirical generalizations.

In conclusion, investigators of phenomena relevant to medical–surgical nursing are generally applying appropriate quantitative methodologies and statistical techniques. However, the application of more sophisticated methods and techniques will enrich research in this area of nursing.

REFERENCES

Bohachick, P. (1984). Progressive relaxation training in cardiac rehabilitation: Effect on psychologic variables. *Nursing Research, 33,* 283–287.

Cohen, J., & Cohen, P. (1975). *Applied multiple regression/correlation analysis for the behavioral sciences.* Hillsdale, NJ: Erlbaum.

Cook, T. D., & Campbell, D. T. (1979). *Quasi-experimentation: Design and analysis of issues in field settings.* Boston: Houghton Mifflin.

Cox, C. L. (1985). The health self-determination index. *Nursing Research, 34,* 177–183.

Dawson, C., Schirmer, M., & Beck, L. (1984). A patient self-disclosure instrument. *Research in Nursing and Health, 7,* 135–147.

Derdiarian, A. K., & Forsythe, A. B. (1983). An instrument for theory and research development using the behavioral systems model for nursing: The cancer patient. *Nursing Research, 32,* 260–166.

Devine, E. C., & Cook, T. D. (1983). A meta-analysis of effects of psychoeducational interventions on length of postsurgical hospital stay. *Nursing Research, 32,* 267–273.

Dickoff, J., & James, P. (1968). A theory of theories: A position paper. *Nursing Research, 17,* 197–203.

Diekman, J. M. (1984). Use of dental irrigating device in the treatment of decubitus ulcers. *Nursing Research, 33,* 303–305.

Dixon, J. (1984). Effects of nursing interventions on nutritional and performance status in cancer patients. *Nursing Research, 33,* 330–335.

Donaldson, S. K., & Crowley, D. M. (1978). The discipline of nursing. *Nursing Outlook, 26,* 113–120.

Dressler, D. K., Smejkal, C., & Ruffolo, M. (1983). A comparison of oral and rectal temperature measurement on patients receiving oxygen by mask. *Nursing Research, 32,* 373–375.

DuCette, J., & Keane, A. (1984). "Why me?": An attributional analysis of major illness. *Research in Nursing and Health, 7,* 257–264.

Fehring, R. J. (1983). Effects of biofeedback-aided relaxation on the psychological stress symptoms of college students. *Nursing Research, 32,* 362–366.

Given, C. W., Given, B. A., Gallin, R. S., & Condon, J. W. (1983). Development of scales to measure beliefs of diabetic patients. *Research in Nursing and Health, 6,* 127–141.

Glass, C. V., McGaw, B., & Smith, M. L. (1981). *Meta-analysis in social research.* Beverly Hills, CA: Sage Publications.

Green, P. E. (1978). *Analyzing multivariate data.* Hinsdale, IL: Dryden.

Harris, R. B., & Hyman, R. B. (1984). Clean vs. sterile tracheotomy care and level of pulmonary infection. *Nursing Research, 33,* 80–85.

Hays, W. L. (1978). *Statistics for the social sciences* (2nd ed.). New York: Holt.

Hubbard, P., Muhlenkamp, A. E., & Brown, N. (1984). The relationship between social support and self-care practices. *Nursing Research, 33,* 266–269.

Jalowiec, A., Murphy, S. P., & Powers, M. J. (1984). Psychometric assessment of the Jalowiec coping scale. *Nursing Research, 33,* 157–161.

Kerlinger, F. N. (1973). *Foundations of behavioral research.* New York: Holt.

Kirchoff, K. T., Rebenson-Piano, M., & Patel, M. K. (1984). Mean arterial pressure readings: Variations with positions and transducer level. *Nursing Research, 33,* 343–345.

Kirk, R. E. (1968). *Experimental design: Procedures for the behavioral sciences.* Belmont, CA: Brooks/Cole.

LeSage, J. (1984). Color vision testing to assist in diagnosis of digoxin toxicity. *Nursing Research, 33,* 346–351.

Levesque, L., Grenier, R., Kerovac, S., & Reidy, M. (1984). Evaluation of a presurgical group program given at two different times. *Research in Nursing and Health, 7,* 227–236.

Levy, P. S., & Lemeshow, S. (1980). *Sampling for health professionals.* Belmont, CA: Lifetime Learning Publications.

Martyn, P. A., Hansen, B. C., & Jen, K. C. (1984). The effects of parenteral nutrition on food intake and gastric motility. *Nursing Research, 33,* 336–342.

Mishel, M. H. (1984). Perceived uncertainty and stress in illness. *Research in Nursing and Health, 7,* 163–171.

Munhall, P. L. (1981). Nursing philosophy and nursing research: In apposition or opposition? *Nursing Research, 30,* 176–177, 181.

Murphy, S. A. (1984). Stress levels and health status of victims of a natural disaster. *Research in Nursing and Health, 7,* 205–215.

O'Connor, A. M. (1983). Factors related to the early phase of rehabilitation following aortocoronary bypass surgery. *Research in Nursing and Health, 6,* 107–116.

Padilla, G. V., Presant, C., Grant, M. M., Metter, G., Lipsett, J., & Heide, F. (1983). Quality of life index for patients with cancer. *Research in Nursing and Health, 6,* 117–126.

Parsons, L. C., & Wilson, M. M. (1984). Cerebrovascular status of severe closed head injured patients following passive position changes. *Nursing Research, 33,* 68–75.

Pedhazur, E. J. (1982). *Multiple regression in behavioral research: Explanation and prediction.* New York: Holt.

Penckoffer, S. H., & Holm, K. (1984). Early appraisal of coronary revascularization on quality of life. *Nursing Research, 33,* 60–63.

Rao, C. R. (1966). Covariance adjustment and related problems in multivariate analysis. In P. R. Krishnaiah (Ed.), *Multivariate analysis* (pp. 87–103). Orlando, FL: Academic Press.

Reynolds, P. D. (1971). *A primer in theory construction.* Indianapolis: Bobbs-Merrill.

Rice, V. H., & Johnson, J. E. (1984). Preadmission self-instruction booklets, postadmission exercise performance, and teaching time. *Nursing Research, 33,* 147–151.

Scott, D. W., Oberst, M. T., & Bookbinder, M. I. (1984). Stress-coping response to genitourinary carcinoma in men. *Nursing Research, 33,* 325–329.

Sexton, D. L., & Munro, B. H. (1985). Impact of a husband's chronic illness (COPD) on the spouses' life. *Research in Nursing and Health, 8,* 83–90.

Sime, S. M., & Libera, M. B. (1985). Sensation information: Self-instruction and responses to dental surgery. *Research in Nursing and Health, 8,* 41–71.

Sitzman, J., Kamuja, J., & Johnston, J. (1983). Biofeedback training for reduced respiratory rate in chronic obstructive pulmonary disease: A preliminary study. *Nursing Research, 32,* 218–223.

Thomas, S. A., Friedmann, E., Lottes, L. S., Gresty, S., Miller, C., & Lynch, J. J. (1984). Changes in nurses' blood pressure and heart rate while communicating. *Research in Nursing and Health, 7,* 119–126.

Vanbree, N. S., Hollerbach, A. D., & Brooks, C. B. (1984). Clinical evaluation of three techniques for administering low-dose heparin. *Nursing Research, 33, 15–19.*

Ventura, M. R., Young, D. E., Feldman, M. J., Pastore, P., Pikula, S., & Yates, M. A. (1984). Effectiveness of health promotion interventions. *Nursing Research, 33,* 162–167.

Wells, P., & Giden, E. (1984). Paraplegic body-support pressure on convoluted foam, waterbed, and standard mattress. *Research in Nursing and Health, 7,* 127–133.

Winer, B. J. (1971). *Statistical principles in experimental design.* New York: McGraw-Hill.

Winslow, E. H., Lane, L. D., & Caffney, F. A. (1985). Oxygen uptake and cardiovascular responses in control adults and acute myocardial infarction patients during bathing. *Nursing Research, 34,* 164–169.

Ziemer, M. M. (1983). Effects of information on postsurgical coping. *Nursing Research, 32,* 282–287.

Comment

Toward Methodological Proficiency in Medical–Surgical Nursing Research

NANCY KLINE LEIDY, Ph.D., R.N.

The preceding chapter provided an excellent overview and critique of the research designs and quantitative methods recently employed in medical–surgical nursing research. Several methodological trends were observed that seemed to denote a blossoming of sophistication in the conduct of quantitative analyses, and insightful recommendations for strengthening empiricism within the profession were made. A few additional observations are offered to stimulate further thought and discussion.

The fundamental purpose of research is to develop theories that describe the interrelationships between concepts and to evaluate their congruency with empirical findings. In 1957, von Mises offered a similar characterization, stating that the purpose of science is "to bring order into the multiplicity of observed phenomena, to predict the course of their development, and to point out ways by which we may bring about the particular phenomena in which we are interested" (p. 7). Theory is the foundation upon which research is built and statistical techniques are merely tools of thought, or intellectual "servants in the investigation of ideas" (Kaplan, 1963, p. 257). Quantitative methods are employed by investigators because they are needed to organize the calculations of inquiry. They do not, and cannot, determine the phenomena to which the calculations are applied, nor what is to be done with the information gained (Kaplan, 1963). These matters represent the essence of research and are the heart of a nurse investigator's practice.

Many of the methodological limitations identified in the preceding chapter reflect a general tendency in nursing to consider the use of empirical methods (i.e., research design and statistical tests) as a primary goal, rather than the means by which theoretically based propositions are examined and tested. Statistics seem to hold a certain mystique across all disciplines. This is particularly true in nursing, however, where the consistent and supported use of empiricism has been relatively recent. Unfortunately, nursing's empirical naiveté is often reflected in the inappropriate application of research methods and statistical models. Furthermore, erroneous techniques are often inadvertently concealed in research reports, through the use of obscure, though seemingly impressive, empirical jargon. It is of utmost importance, therefore, that we outgrow this developmental stage of methodological idolatry by acquiring higher levels of proficiency in the use of research design and quantitative analysis.

The call for the use of more sophisticated quantitative methods in nursing research is justified. It is important to note, however, that it is not the complexity of the statistic per se that is the issue. As previously stated, statistics are only instruments by which theoretical formulations are tested. It is the appropriate use of statistical methods that should be of primary concern. Developing greater sophistication in medical-surgical nursing research should not necessarily be equated with the use of more complex mathematical models. Rather, methodological proficiency should be measured by the consistently appropriate use of a wide variety of empirical tools to answer theoretically based questions.

With this goal of proficiency in mind, let us outline and discuss several of the misrepresentations and misapplications observed in the medical-surgical nursing research literature, as stated in the preceding chapter.

1. *The inappropriate application of multiple comparison tests, most commonly post hoc comparison and multiple t-tests, when fixed-effects analysis of variance (ANOVA) was employed.* Clearly, the results from multiple *t*-tests will be biased, because the probabil-

ity of falsely rejecting at least one null hypothesis will increase as the number of t-tests conducted increases. For simple pairwise comparisons of means among samples of equal size, Tukey's multiple-comparison method is a more powerful tool. In situations involving unequal sample sizes or where contrasts, rather than pairwise comparisons, are of primary interest, Scheffe's method is preferred (Kleinbaum & Kupper, 1978).

2. *Failure to report testing for the homogeneity of regression assumption when analysis of covariance was applied to the data.* It is difficult to ascertain whether this situation involves (a) a failure on the part of the investigators to explore their data fully; (b) a failure to report this exploration; or (c) a preference by the editors to assume this testing had been done and to eliminate unnecessary detail from the manuscript. The need to include detailed accounts of statistical tests in published manuscripts is controversial. It is unfortunate, however, that we cannot yet assume that appropriate prerequisite data explorations are done before statistical tests are applied and results are reported.

3. *Failure to explore interaction effects adequately in the multiple-factor analysis of variance.* It is important to recall that when two factors interact, there is some question as to the true meaning of factor level measures. Interactions may be so important that effects should not even be addressed in terms of factor level means. Conversely, interactions may be unimportant, or so nearly parallel that for all practical purposes, analysis of factor effects can proceed as though no interaction exists (Neter & Wasserman, 1974). Full exploration of interaction is particularly important for nursing intervention studies where these effects have important practice implications.

4. *Inappropriate use of multiple univariate techniques rather than multivariate analyses.* In this situation, the tendency to use repeated analysis of variance (ANOVA) techniques rather than the preferred multivariate analysis of variance (MANOVA) approach was noted. Goodwin (1984) also found occasions in nursing research when multiple single-factor ANOVAs were applied rather than a factorial ANOVA and when simple correlational analyses were employed rather than a multiple regression analysis. The potential and appropriate use of multivariate statistics should be examined further.

5. *Inappropriate selection of parametric tests when levels of measurement were ordinal or nominal, rather than continuous.* It is important to note that this objection is controversial. Many investigators and statisticians feel it is quite appropriate to treat

ordinal data as interval-level data (Henry, 1982; Kim, 1975; Labovitz, 1967, 1970, 1971, 1972; Mayer, 1970, 1971; O'Brien, 1979).

6. *Failure to use randomization in the selection or assignment of subjects, and the use of a quasi-experimental design in such situations.* Unfortunately, the problems of nonrandomization cannot be overcome simply by labeling a study "quasi-experimental." Furthermore, the general failure to utilize some form of random sampling technique is compounded by a tendency to employ relatively small sample sizes in nursing research. These limitations have dramatic implications for the application of probability theory, whose principle of randomness lies at the heart of statistical methods. Nursing must attempt to resolve this dilemma through the use of creative subject recruitment strategies and more rigorous sampling techniques.

Until methodological difficulties such as these are overcome, the capacity to draw inferences and build nursing knowledge is compromised. Thus, efforts should be directed toward increasing knowledge and expanding proficiency in the application of statistical methods commonly used in medical–surgical nursing research. Nursing's investigative knowledge base must include a thorough understanding of the mathematical models, assumptions, and limitations of different statistical models.

The recommendation that the nursing profession continue to build its knowledge base through the conduct of descriptive and exploratory research should be endorsed emphatically. Such empirical efforts will contribute to the identification and understanding of the innumerable physiological, psychological, and social phenomena involved in the processes of health and illness. The development of newly identified constructs of relevance to nursing practice entails factor-isolating and factor-relating levels of theory development (Dickoff, James, & Wiedenbach, 1968). These theoretical approaches, by their very nature, compel investigators to employ descriptive and exploratory research designs. The new constructs will mature through a cyclical process that will ultimately encompass all levels of theory development and require more diverse empirical designs and analytical techniques.

However, it is also true that research problems derived from factor-relating, situation-relating, and prescriptive levels of theory development are already prevalent in the nursing literature. It is therefore mandatory that we develop proficiency in the application of a wider variety of quantitative methods and become knowledgeable in statistical techniques that are more appropriate to these problems. Causal modeling, for example, was identified by Roberts as an important instrument for the exploration of nursing phenomena. It is important to note that the success of causal modeling is dependent upon the existence of valid and reliable construct indicators, appropriate data collection techniques, and accurate use of data reduction strategies. Once again, we must rely heavily upon the appropriate application of quantitative methods at all levels of analysis in order to insure accuracy in nursing's database.

Meta-analysis is another important and highly relevant statistical model for nursing research. This technique, when used appropriately, will enable us to synthesize information from numerous research reports and determine average treatment effects and treatment variability from replication to replication (Carlberg & Miller, 1984). This will prove to be exceedingly helpful in understanding and validating empirically the effectiveness of nursing interventions. To take full advantage of this technique, particularly in light of the small sample sizes prevalent in nursing research, replication should be encouraged. The use of meta-analysis will also require that appropriate consideration be given to the procedure's parametric and stochastic assumptions (Abraham & Schultz, 1983).

In summary, it is of utmost importance that nurse investigators continue to develop greater proficiency in the application of commonly employed research designs and quantitative methods. As we develop this proficiency, we must also begin to expand our intellectual efforts to include the exploration of "new" mathematical tools that will enable investigators to address more adequately the increasingly complex theoretical concerns and empirical issues involved in nursing research.

REFERENCES

Abraham, I. L., & Schultz, S. (1983). Univariate statistical models for meta-analysis. *Nursing Research, 32,* 312–315.

Carlberg, C. G., & Miller, T. L. (1984). Introduction to the special issue on meta-analysis. *Journal of Special Education, 18,* 9–10.

Dickoff, J., James, P., & Wiedenbach, E. (1968). Theory in a practice discipline. *Nursing Research, 17,* 415–435.

Goodwin, L. D. (1984). Increasing efficiency and precision of data analysis: Multivariate vs. univariate statistical techniques. *Nursing Research, 33*, 247–249.

Henry, F. (1982). Multivariate analysis and ordinal data. *American Sociological Review, 47*, 299–304.

Kaplan, A. (1963). *The conduct of inquiry*. Scranton, PA: Chandler.

Kim, J. O. (1975). Multivariate analysis of ordinal variables. *American Journal of Sociology, 84*, 448–456.

Kleinbaum, D. G., & Kupper, L. L. (1978). *Applied regression analysis and other multivariable methods*. Boston: Duxbury.

Labovitz, S. (1967). Some observations on measurement and statistics. *Social Forces, 46*, 151–160.

Labovitz, S. (1970). The assignment of numbers to rank order categories. *American Sociological Review, 35*, 515–524.

Labovitz, S. (1971). In defense of assigning numbers to ranks. *American Sociological Review, 36*, 521–522.

Labovitz, S. (1972). Statistical usage in sociology: Sacred cows and ritual. *Sociological Methods and Research, 1*, 13–37.

Mayer, L. S. (1970). Comments on "The assignment of numbers to rank order categories." *American Sociological Review, 35*, 916–917.

Mayer, L. S. (1971). A note on treating ordinal data as interval data. *American Sociological Review, 36*, 519–520.

Mises, R. von. (1957). *Probability, statistics, and truth*. New York: Dover.

Neter, J., & Wasserman, W. (1974). *Applied linear statistical models*. Homewood, IL: Irwin.

O'Brien, R. M. (1979). The use of Pearson's R with ordinal data. *American Sociological Review, 44*, 851–857.

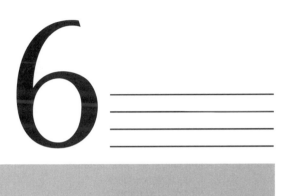

Statistics and Quantitative Research Methods in Nursing Care of Children

MARIE L. LOBO, Ph.D., R.N.
KATHLEEN ROSS-ALAOLMOLKI, Ph.D., R.N.

This chapter presents a comprehensive review and analysis of published nursing research related to children, as well as suggestions for the future of research in this domain of nursing. Identifying the boundaries for inclusion and exclusion in this review was certainly a challenge. For instance, it was difficult to define and delineate the characteristics of the studies to be included in our review. We decided to limit the review to studies in which the data were obtained directly from the child. This eliminated studies that surveyed parents only, for parent data may not convey what is really happening with the child. Similarly, studies with data provided by nurses about children were omitted. In addition, there were some studies in which it was unclear whether the source of data was the child or the adult, and these studies were excluded as well. Finally, we did not consider studies done by nonnurses but presented in the nursing literature. We recognize the potential controversy of this decision.

The difficulties in deciding about the admissibility of certain studies to this review were compounded by a lack of clarity concerning research methodology found in many reports. Many studies had nonexistent or poorly stated conceptual and operational definitions. Descriptions of instruments often did not include information on their psychometric properties, especially those that were developed by the investigators for the specific purpose of the study. Often the appropriateness of statistical tests was difficult to evaluate.

We surveyed all issues of *Nursing Research, Research in Nursing and Health, American Journal of Maternal Child Nursing, Advances in Nursing Science,* and *Topics in Clinical Nursing. Pediatric Nursing* and *Maternal Child Nursing Journal* were reviewed where applicable.

Review of Published Research

Studies were reviewed in relationship to four major areas: design, sample size, measurement, and statistical analysis.

DESIGN

Descriptive Research. Descriptive research has as its "main objective the accurate portrayal of the characteristics of persons, situations, or groups, and the frequency with which certain phenomena occur" (Polit & Hungler, 1983, p. 613). Thirty-nine studies were descriptive. The sample sizes in these studies varied from 3 to 986. Some of these studies were retrospective, although generally very few retrospective studies were reported in the literature.

Correlational Research. The second type of design to be discussed is a variation of purely descriptive research and is termed *correlational research.* This includes "investigations that explore the interrelationships among variables of interest without any active intervention on the part of the researcher" (Polit & Hungler, 1983, p. 612). Thirteen studies were reviewed that described relationships between two or more events. The sample sizes in these studies ranged from 18 to 193. A few studies were retrospective. Since nurses are said to be interested in the associative relationships of various phenomena, it was surprising that not more correlational studies emerged from the literature.

Experimental and Quasi-Experimental Research. Experimental research consists of investigations in which the "investigator manipulates the independent variable and randomly assigns subjects to different conditions" (Polit & Hungler, 1983, p. 613). Quasi-experimental research includes studies "in which subjects cannot be randomly assigned to treatment conditions, although the research does manipulate the independent variable and exercises certain controls to enhance the internal validity of the results" (Polit & Hungler, 1983, p. 620). We identified twenty-three studies that were experimental or quasi-experimental with sample sizes ranging from 5 to 4316.

Instrument Development. Five studies were focused on the development of instruments for use with children. These studies had sample sizes between 14 and 940.

Case Studies. Only one study retained for this review was a case study, although we encountered a number of them in the literature.

SAMPLE SIZE

The studies included in the review had sample sizes ranging from one (in the case study report) to well over 4000 in a study on decreasing the negative effects of mass inoculation on children in Minnesota (Hedburg & Schlong, 1973). It was noted that, considering the sample size, inappropriate statistics were used at times. This was particularly true in experimental and quasi-experimental studies, many of which were exploratory, although they were not labeled as such.

MEASUREMENT

Structured Observation. The most frequent measurement technique was structured observation of the child, with 26 studies employing this technique. Of these, seven included observation of both child and parent in an interaction context. The technique of structured observation involves the investigator or the research assistant watching the child and recording specific behaviors from a predetermined list of defined behaviors. Many studies included in our review lacked information on interobserver reliability and on standardization of the definitions of the behaviors being observed.

Unstructured Observation. Eight studies employed unstructured observation of children's behaviors. These studies were plagued by many problems. Often the definitions of behaviors were unclear or nonexistent. There was little information about interobserver reliability or any attempt to standardize the observations. At times, assumptions were not articulated. It must be noted that some of these studies were solely exploratory in nature.

Questionnaires. Fourteen studies used questionnaires on children for purposes of data collection. These studies almost invariably involved school-aged children or adolescents. The reading and comprehension skills necessary to complete the questionnaires were rarely discussed in the research reports.

Biophysical Measures. Measures of a biophysical nature (e.g., blood pressure, pulse, and temperature) were used in 19 studies. The reliability of the instrument used was discussed consistently across most studies. Biophysical measures were used most prominently in hospitalized children or children about to undergo a clinical procedure. In some studies, the report of the biophysical measures was taken from the chart and integrated with additional data collected from other sources or with other techniques.

Chart Review. Chart or record review data were reported in 14 studies. These data were often added to other data obtained directly from the child. It was noted that studies gave little attention to the reliability of these data, the inherent assumption being that health care providers record data accurately in the first place.

Interviews: Structured and Unstructured. In 11 studies data were collected from structured interviews, and in five studies the data were from unstructured interviews. Five studies also involved combined parent–child interviews, and in one study a physician was interviewed as well. There was great variability in data collection methods and in the reporting of reliability and validity information. The preparation of the interviewer was rarely discussed, and little consideration was given to the potential for recorder bias.

Play as a method of interview data collection was used in three studies and involved recordings of children's behaviors and statements during a play experience. The interpretations and evaluations of these recordings were often very subjective, and interrater reliability was seldom reported. None of the studies involved videotaping play situations.

Standardized interviewing methods were used in 16 studies. The credentials of the individual or individuals administering the test were rarely addressed. Although the quality of an environment is often important in the reliable use of standardized interviewing protocols, descriptions of environment were most often lacking. We also found four studies in which data were collected through drawing or projective techniques.

STATISTICAL ANALYSIS

Evaluating the statistical techniques applied in the studies was a challenging task, mainly because of the poor quality of some of the studies or the lack of pertinent information in many of the reports.

Descriptive Statistics. All the studies used frequencies to describe part or all of the data. Forty-eight studies inappropriately drew extensive conclusions or interpretations from these frequencies. Further, 22 studies used the mean and 10 studies used the standard deviation to give meaning to data. Percentages were found in 11 reports. Interestingly, 10 relied only on descriptive statistics and based all their conclusions on these parameters.

Chi-square. We found 16 studies in which the chi-square test was applied to nominal variables. Although this test was rarely misused, several studies could have been strengthened if a more powerful statistic had been employed.

Analysis of Variance. Analysis of variance models governed the data analysis of 15 investigations. It was not always indicated which ANOVA model was being applied. In three studies, one-way ANOVA was used, with two-way ANOVA found in another three studies. Several of these studies had measurements over time, yet often it was unclear whether a repeated-measures ANOVA was used in the statistical analysis.

Multivariate Analysis. Multivariate analyses such as regression analysis (which, admittedly, can also be argued to be a univariate method), multivariate analysis of variance, and factor analysis were reported in 15 articles. Studies using these techniques tended to have more sophisticated designs and data collection procedures than did many of the other studies in our review. Most of the investigations were done in the 1970s and the 1980s, and the use of advanced statistics is a reflection of the increasing sophistication of nursing research.

T-test. The *t*-test was used to test for differences in means in 25 of the reports, including five studies in which the statistical test was not specified but most likely was a *t*-test. Often parameters were not specified, the type of *t*-test not stated, and the issue of homogeneity of variances not discussed.

Nonparametric Statistics. Eight studies used nonparametric methods, including the Mann-Whitney U, the Wilcoxon Matched Pairs test, and the Kolmogorov-Smirnov test. These tests were all used appropriately with the appropriate sample size and appropriate level of measurement.

Qualitative Analysis. The data analysis of nine studies had some elements of qualitative analysis. In some cases they included the frequency with which a topic was mentioned in an interview or with which a behavior was noted. Often meanings were attributed to such frequencies or to statements made by subjects, especially if some intervention had been implemented.

Quality of Current Research

Considering the preceding findings, it is reasonable to state that the quality of the research reported in the literature of the nursing care of children is variable at best. A few issues can be identified in this regard.

Particularly striking is that only two *programs* of research could be identified in the domain of nursing care of children. The first is the sequence of studies on suck in the neonate by Anderson and her associates (Anderson, McBride, Dahm, Ellis, & Vidyasagar, 1982; Burroughes, Asonya, Anderson-Shanklin, & Vedyasagar, 1978; Ellison, Vidyasagar, & Anderson, 1979; Measel & Anderson, 1979). The second program of study is presented in the work of Barnard and her associates, which reflects a 15-year program of inquiry (Barnard, 1973, 1985; Barnard, Bee, & Hammond, 1984; Barnard, Booth, Mitchell, & Telgrow, 1982; Barnard & Eyres, 1979; Eyres, Barnard, & Gray, 1979). In contrast to these two programs of research, individual investigators have studied selected topics without concern about the creation of a systematic body of knowledge about nursing care of children.

This brings up the issue of scientific mentorship, and more specifically, the current scarcity of mentors for new researchers. This scarcity is problematic in that inexperienced researchers often need assistance in accessing and mastering complex academic and health care systems to implement their research. The lack of role models for new investigators also hinders the development of new programs of research, let alone the maturation of these investigators themselves.

We also noted gaps in research on children with certain underlying health conditions. This problem is particularly pertinent in the area of chronic illness. The majority of the research on children with chronic illness has been done from the parent's perspective and mostly with only maternal input. This may result from the belief that these children need to be protected from researchers or from the assumption that children cannot give valid responses. In reality, children as young as six years of age can understand the concept of consent and can determine whether they should participate in research projects (Weithorn, 1983).

Directions for the Future

From our review of research on nursing care of children a number of recommendations for research development in this area can be formulated. The major suggestion we wish to make is the need for the development of systematic programs of inquiry. These programs should include both descriptive investigations and experimental and quasi-experimental ones. The descriptive aspects of a program of research can become the basis for the interventions of the future. When coupled with the wealth of data available in both the clinical and research literature, investigations that test nursing interventions in a systematic manner can be developed. More generally, there is a continued need for more experimental and quasi-experimental research.

We also argue for the integration of time series designs in this research effort. The focus of the discipline of nursing is on the responses of the individual in a state of health or illness. These states do not appear in isolation, yet they occur through time and space and are dynamic. To measure these phenomena at a single data collection point is a disservice to pediatric nursing.

There is a strong emphasis in nursing research on studies with large sample sizes that conform to principles of statistical power analysis. However, it must be acknowledged that not all future investigations in the area of nursing care of children will have these desirable large sample sizes. In fact, the requisite for such samples may place great burdens on the investigators. Children with specific health problems are often difficult to access in large numbers. When they are accessible, they are often "protected" from researchers by well-meaning adults. Healthy children in school systems are also protected, in this case by the regulations of the respective school districts. Although we advocate the protection of children from unnecessary investigations, it should be recognized that excessive and undue concern may result in an increasingly difficult environment for research on children. It should also be added that, when investigations are done with small sample sizes, the appropriate statistical procedures should be applied.

The case study approach is a type of investigation that should receive more consideration. Barnard (1983) has discussed the need for using this approach as a research tool to enhance the knowledge base in nursing.

Research on nursing care of children will also be enriched if clinical trials of nursing interventions are implemented. The integration of clinical trials with other types of research will ultimately lead to the establishment of a repertoire of clinical interventions with children of all age groups.

There is a need to use more powerful statistics in research in pediatric nursing. However, it must be stressed that these statistics must be appropriate to the design and methods of the investigation. Multivariate statistics should be used more extensively to understand better the many factors influencing children's health and well-being. The use of a multivariate approach to problems in nursing care of children is, in our opinion, a critical factor in the development of a knowledge base in the field.

Finally, to develop a theoretical basis for nursing of children as discussed previously, we propose that research be centered around children's responses to a health problem and the environment. We favor a systematic building of a knowledge base around the core concepts of health, human responses, environment, and nursing interventions and believe that thus a body of knowledge about nursing care of children may evolve.

REFERENCES

Anderson, G. C., McBride, M. R., Dahm, J., Ellis, M. K., & Vidyasagar, D. (1982). Development of sucking in term infants from birth to four hours postbirth. *Research in Nursing and Health, 5*, 21–27.

Barnard, K. B. (1973). The effect of stimulation on sleep. *Behavior of the Premature Infant, 6,* 12–33.

Barnard, K. (1983). MCN keys to research: The case study method: A research tool. *American Journal of Maternal Child Nursing, 8,* 36.

Barnard, K. E., (1985). Nursing systems towards effective parenting—Premature. *Final Report.* Seattle: University of Washington.

Barnard, K. E., & Eyres, S. J. (Eds.) (1979). *Child Health Assessment Part 2: The first year of life.* DHEW Publication No. HRA 79–25. Hyattsville, MD: U.S. Department of Health, Education, and Welfare.

Barnard, K. E., Booth, C. L., Mitchell, S. K., & Telzrow, R. W. (1982). *Newborn nursing models.* Final report of project RO1-NUOO719, DHHS, HRA, BHMP, Division of Nursing. Seattle: Department of Parent and Child Nursing, School of Nursing, University of Washington.

Barnard, K. E., Bee, H. L., Hammond, M. A. (1984). Home environment and cognitive development in a healthy, low-risk sample: The Seattle study. In A.W. Gottfried (Ed.), *Home environment and early cognitive development longitudinal research* (pp. 117–149). Orlando, FL: Academic Press.

Burroughes, A. K., Asonye, U. O., Anderson-Shanklin, G. C., & Vidyasagar D. (1978). The effect of nonnutrition sucking on transcutaneous oxygen tension in noncrying preterm neonates. *Research in Nursing and Health, 1,* 69–75.

Ellison, S. L., Vidyasagar, D., & Anderson, G. C. (1979). Sucking in the newborn infant during the first hour of life. *Journal of Nurse Midwifery,* 18–25.

Eyres, S. J., Barnard, K. E., & Gray, C. A. (1979). *Child health assessment: Part III 2-4 years.* Final report of project RO2-NUOO559, DHHS, HRA, BHMP, Division of Nursing. Seattle: Maternal and Child Nursing Department, School of Nursing, University of Washington.

Hedburg, A. G., & Schlong, A. (1973). Eliminating fainting by school children during mass inoculation clinics. *Nursing Research, 22,* 352–353.

Measel, C. P., & Anderson, G. C. (1979). Nonnutritive sucking during tube feedings: Effect on clinical course in premature infants. *Journal of Obstetrical and Gynecological Nursing, 8,* 265–272.

Polit, D. F., & Hungler, B. P. (1983). *Nursing research: Principles and methods.* Philadelphia: Lippincott.

Weithorn, L. A. (1983). Children's capacities to decide about participation in research. *IRA: A Review of Human Subject Research* 5(2), 1–5.

Comment

Implications for Design, Sampling, Measurement, and Statistical Analysis in Parent–Child Nursing Research

HEIDI VONKOSS KROWCHUK, Ph.D., R.N.

The preceding chapter alludes to a number of potentially important aspects of nursing of children research that will further research in this domain of nursing. By explicating and elaborating these aspects it is possible to address the implications for design, sampling, measurement, and statistical analysis of the findings reported in the chapter.

Design

The survey of the research literature revealed that a variety of methods have been used to investigate phenomena within the nursing of children domain and that the most prevalent designs were descriptive, followed by experimental and quasi-experimental. This is consistent with the findings of Brown, Tanner, and Padrick (1984). In a content analysis of nursing research articles published from 1952 to 1980, these authors found that the largest proportion of studies claimed description as their goal.

Interestingly, Brown et al. (1984) noticed a shift away from descriptive studies over the past three decades to an increase in explanatory studies. Jacobson and Meininger (1985) analyzed the designs and methods used in published nursing research from 1956 to 1983. The results of this analysis verified the findings of Brown et al. (1984) of a trend in published research that moves away from description and toward explanation. It is possible to interpret this change in research focus as an indication of increased research sophisticaton among investigators and increased versatility in the methods of science. This is certainly evident in the nursing of children research literature.

A paucity of methodological studies in the pediatric nursing literature was noted and is cause for concern. The few methodological studies encountered were concerned solely with instrument development. A priority in nursing of children research is the need to develop instruments to be used by nurses to index behavior and interaction patterns of children, parents, nurses, and health care systems. The development and availability of credible measures will advance the testing of theoretical formulations underlying the practice of nursing of children. Linked to this is the need to examine the specific realities of nursing research within the parent–child field (e.g., problems related to access to subjects, the continuing development of the child, etc.) in order to develop methods, designs, and statistical paradigms that address these realities and problems.

Case studies, valuable to nursing practice because they allow for the recording of changes in clients and their individual responses to treatment when large samples are not available or practical, continue to be used infrequently. In advocating the use of the case study method, it is important to consider the use of a common framework for structuring the reporting of case studies. Use of a common structure would foster an accumulation of knowledge regarding child responses to health problems and nursing interventions. This knowledge could be used to identify further areas for nursing research.

Sampling

Sample sizes varied from study to study, and it may indeed be that small sample sizes are unavoidable because of the problems encountered in accessing large numbers of children to serve as subjects in research projects. Although it may be that well-meaning adults protect children from nurse researchers, another reason for this problem seems to stem from the informed consent procedures with which investigators must comply in doing research on child subjects. In research on adults using the techniques of interview or questionnaire, consent to participate is assumed if the subject agrees to complete a questionnaire or answers questions in an interview. To protect children's rights, both the child's assent and the parent's permission are required. This is necessary because children may not be capable of recognizing that their responses to questions on sensitive issues may be potentially damaging to themselves or others (Department of Health and Human Services, 1983). This regulation continues to be as vital as ever to ensure the protection of children involved as research subjects. However, it also places an additional responsibility on the investigator in that an explanation of the study must be provided to the child within the framework of the child's comprehension. This can become problematic when the potential child subject, from whom the investigator wishes to obtain assent, is younger than school age.

The difficulty of adhering to normative models for sampling in conducting research on clinical problems in children is pertinent. Subjects tend to be few in number and are usually not selected in a truly random manner from the entire population of potential subjects. Similarly, in both experimental and quasi-experimental designs, the possibility of a comparison or control group is desirable. In many instances a random control group that has all the characteristics of the referent population is difficult to obtain. Matched sample, cohort, and blocked designs, as well as latin-squares and greco-latin squares, are designs that are not often used in parent–child nursing research, but that certainly could serve as potential solutions to sampling problems (Kirk, 1982).

Measurement

Variables of interest are measured in numerous ways in nursing care of children research. However, a recurrent problem is that seldom are the psychometric or other characteristics reported. This has been noted in the nursing literature at large (Batey, 1977; Brown et al., 1984; Jacobsen & Meininger, 1985). The inclusion of reliability and validity data in research reports is esssential, especially since some instruments used by nurse researchers were developed in other disciplines and often only loosely correspond to the conceptual meanings of the variables of interest.

A related measurement issue has to do with construct validity of presumed causes and effects, which refers to inferences made about abstract constructs; e.g., cause, reliable change, and reliable differences (Cook & Campbell, 1979). In nursing care of children, studies often pertain to changes, differences, and their causes, yet seldom do we see reports on the threats to construct validity that may be present in these studies.

Statistical Analysis

Given that descriptive studies were found to be the primary method of inquiry, it is not surprising that descriptive statistics predominated. Yet, as pointed out in the preceding chapter, we can see a progression in the sophistication of data analyses. Multivariate analysis is beginning to appear in research on nursing care of children. It can be expected that multivariate studies, which examine the interrelations among a broad array of variables, will soon dominate the literature (Lederman, 1984). Only by applying the findings from such studies can a systematic and cumulative testing of relationships proceed, and thus achieve understanding of complex nursing problems.

Conclusion

The preceding chapter perhaps creates the impression that the accumulated knowledge base in the area of nursing care of children is tenuous and fragmented. These concerns seems to be common to all specialty areas of nursing, and many of the chapters in this book provide evidence to that effect. The research is essentially noncumulative. Often it is not linked to prior work, or it does not appear to be planned so as to clarify, advance, or refute theoretical or conceptual formulations (Batey, 1977; Denyes, 1983; Fawcett, 1984; Gortner, 1980; Haller, Reynolds, &

Horsley, 1979). Indeed, only through the development of systematic programs of research will conceptual clustering of studies be promoted. In turn, this will advance the knowledge base within the nursing of children domain.

The preceding chapter offers methodological suggestions for strenthening the body of knowledge about nursing care of children, including the use of time series designs, clinical trials, and experimental and quasi-experimental methods. Although by themselves these suggestions are valid, we also need the theory that helps us predict and control outcomes. Moreover, these methods may not always be feasible or economical. This is not to say that our research should be inferior because of logistics or cost, yet it is important to balance these different factors. Consequently, it is likely that descriptive and correlational studies will still be conducted in an effort to describe phenomena of interest and their interrelationships. The nature of the questions asked and the phenomena to be studied should mandate the method for study rather than the method being the determinant (Ellis, 1982).

REFERENCES

Barnard, K. (1983). MCN keys to research: The case study method. *American Journal of Maternal Child Nursing, 8*, 36.

Batey, M. (1977). Conceptualization: Knowledge and logic guiding empirical research. *Nursing Research, 26*, 324–329.

Brown, J., Tanner, C., & Padrick, K. (1984). Nursing's search for scientific knowledge. *Nursing Research, 33*, 26–32.

Cook, T., & Campbell, D. (1979). *Quasi-experimental: Design & analysis issues for field settings*. Boston: Houghton Mifflin Company.

Denyes, M. (1983). Nursing research related to schoolage children and adolescents. *Annual Review of Nursing Research, 1*, 27–53.

Department of Health and Human Services (1983). Additional protection for children involved as subjects in research. *Federal Register, 48*, 9814–9820.

Ellis, R. (1982). Editorial. *Advances in Nursing Science, 4*(4), x–xi.

Fawcett, J. (1984). The metaparadigm of nursing: Present status and future refinements. *Image: The Journal of Nursing Scholarship, 16*, 84–89.

Gortner, S. (1980). Nursing Science in transition. *Nursing Research, 29*, 180–183.

Haller, K., Reynolds, M., & Horsley, J. (1979). Developing research-based innovation protocols: Process, criteria and issues. *Research in Nursing and Health, 2*, 45–51.

Jacobsen, B., & Meininger, J. (1985). The designs and methods of published nursing research: 1956–1983. *Nursing Research, 34*, 306–312.

Kirk, R. (1982). *Experimental design: Procedures for the behavioral sciences*. Belmont, CA: Brooks/Cole Publishing Company.

Lederman, R. (1984). Anxiety and conflict in pregnancy: Relationship to maternal health status. *Annual Review of Nursing Research, 2*, 27–62.

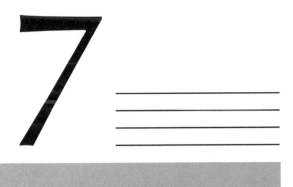

Women's Health Research: Implications for Design, Measurement, and Analysis

MARTHA LENTZ, Ph.D., R.N.
NANCY FUGATE WOODS, Ph.D., R.N., F.A.A.N.

The women's health movement, part of the feminist movement of the 1960s, fostered critical analysis of women's health services, professional literature dealing with women and their health, and common practices of health professionals. Critical analysis of the professional literature revealed an astounding lack of knowledge about women and their health. Most research conducted prior to the 1970s focused on women as childbearers and childrearers and on reproductive system disorders. Since the early 1970s there has been an increased emphasis on the health of the woman herself. Despite increased emphasis on studying women, there is not yet a clear definition of the field of study called *women's health*.

Definitions

For purposes of our discussion, we define women's health as a field of inquiry, practice, and education. The primary focus of this field is on the health of the woman herself, in contrast to the view of woman as childbearer or childrearer. Emerging work is concerned with psychosocial and physiological well-being of women, with recognition of the interrelationships between women's health and the biological, social, and cultural contexts of women's lives. The following concepts are central to the study of women's health in nursing: women, environment, health, and nursing. *Women* refers to all people of the feminine gender. Because of the continuity of influence and gender on health throughout the lifespan, female children can be included within the scope of women's health scholarship. *Environment* refers to the contexts in which women experience health: the social, cultural, and biophysical milieus. Special environments influencing women's health are the family and organizations. *Health* reflects the woman's feelings of well-being, functional abilities, and experiences of symptoms and health concerns. Health-seeking behavior as well as health status are linked to the concept of women's health. Women's health scholarship addresses:

1. Women's health experiences across the lifespan;
2. The interrelationship between women's health and environment;
3. The process of attaining, retaining, and regaining health as women experience them (Woods, 1988; McBride & McBride, 1981).

Within the discipline of *nursing*, women's health scholarship has a special focus. Nursing practice emphasizes the diagnosis and treatment of human responses to actual and potential health problems. Nursing science includes knowledge about how individuals adapt to wellness and illness; how families cope in health and illness situations such as transitions like birthing, as well as illness-related changes; how the biophysical, psychosocial, and cultural environments affect development and maintenance of health; how physical and interpersonal interventions assist people and their families in reducing the negative consequences of illness; how people cope with the physical, psychological, interpersonal, and social effects of illness; and how health and health-related behaviors can be promoted (Barnard, 1980).

In this chapter we address issues related to nursing research in the area of women's health. We begin with an overview of predominant foci of content and methodologies in this research effort. This is followed by recommendations for nursing science approaches to studying women's health. These recommendations are presented within the context of a current research project.

State of the Science

In 1981, McBride and McBride lamented the lack of attention to women's lived experiences in contemporary women's health research. They called for increased emphasis of women's first-person experiences as embedded in the context of their lives; an approachment of subjective and objective methods; and generation of theoretical frameworks to explain women's health. Women's health research published in nursing journals from 1980 to 1985 (*Journal of Obstetrical and Gynecologic Nursing, Nursing Research, Research in Nursing and Health, Western Journal of Nursing Research, Advances in Nursing Science, Maternal Child Nursing*, and *Health Care of Women International*) does not reflect great progress toward meeting the McBrides' 1981 challenges (Woods, 1988).

The phenomena most frequently addressed in women's health research published in the nursing literature include responses to *transitional states*, such as pregnancy and birth, menarche, and menopause; *health in relation to the environment*, such as studies relating the social environment to depression and symptom formation; *human responses to illness* and treatment of illness, such as adaptation to mastectomy; and *health-seeking behavior*, such as contraceptive practices, weight control attempts, and therapeutic processes to improve health.

Several features are common to these phenomena. First, each is best understood as a *dynamic*, not a static phenomenon. The phenomena themselves change over time, and it is likely that factors associated with the phenomena also change over time. Consider in this regard the inherently dynamic nature of pregnancy, labor and childbirth, menarche, and menopause. Changes in health status occurring in conjunction with environmental change, adaptation to role changes, and responses to stressors characteristic of women's lives each imply the necessity of understanding *process* and evolving *patterns*.

Second, phenomena addressed in women's health research are multidimensional, cutting across the boundaries of traditional disciplines. For example, pregnancy and aging involve biophysical adaptation, changes in the self, changes in role relationships, and changing relationships of the woman to her environment. To achieve a holistic rather than particularistic understanding of these phenomena, research techniques that address multiple dimensions of health are essential.

For the most part, women's health researchers have treated these phenomena as static constructs. Most of the investigators whose papers were published between 1980 and 1985 employed single-occasion measures. The analytic strategies included tests of association and difference. In several cases, multivariate analysis was employed, but in only a few was a causal modeling technique (such as path analysis) used to analyze the presumed sequence of events. When multiple measurements were made, the analytic strategies used (such as analysis of variance for repeated measures) partitioned the variance resulting from sequence of measures but did not characterize a pattern of events as they unfolded over time.

As a rule, the investigators treated the concepts they studied as unidimensional, even though their frameworks often described concepts as multidimensional and reflected consideration of work from several disciplines. Yet most measured the constructs as if influenced by a simple disciplinary perspective (e.g., psychology or sociology), in stark contrast to the richness of the conceptual framework.

Recommendations for Nursing Science Approaches to Studying Women's Health

We recommend that future work reflect the dynamism and patterns in women's health. In particular, we recommend that investigators employ

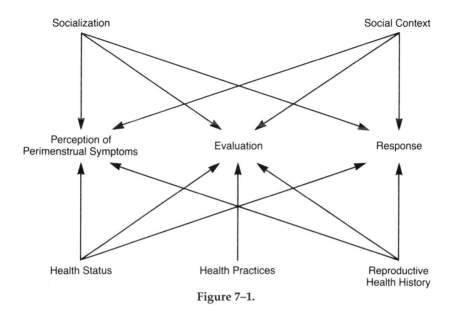

Figure 7–1.

methods that foster understanding of women's health as constantly changing processes. Moreover, we recommend that investigators employ analytic strategies that foster identification of holistic understanding of women's health, reflecting patterns of integration of biological, psychosocial, and cultural components.

In the following discussion we use an ongoing investigation to illustrate some approaches for studying change as transitions or dynamic processes. In addition, we illustrate ways of studying phenomena such as health patterns from a holistic perspective. The study we use to exemplify our points is focused on health-seeking behavior related to perimenstrual symptoms.

The purpose of the study included testing of the model given in Figure 7-1. The health-seeking process is central to this model, with perception of symptoms, evaluation of symptoms, and response to symptoms being the central elements. Perception of symptoms refers to whether the woman notices certain feelings or behaviors during the perimenstruum. Symptom evaluation refers to the judgments the woman makes about her symptoms, such as their severity, treatability, causes, and effects on her life. Response to symptoms refers to the feelings, thoughts, and behaviors that occur as a consequence of symptoms. Based on earlier work with the health-seeking process (Chrisman & Kleinman, 1977), we hypothesize that these components of the process are affected by socialization; the current social milieu, including dimensions of stress and social support; and the woman's own health status, history, and practices.

METHOD

The sampling framework employed in the study involved procedures to ensure representation of women from white, black, and Asian ethnic groups of middle income. Households in the designated neighborhoods were screened to identify eligible women willing to participate in the study. Participants completed an in-home interview and a 90-day health diary. After women completed their diaries, some were asked to participate in a food diary. These women also completed a telephone interview.

MEASURES

The model has three components of the health-seeking process: perception of symptoms, evaluation of symptoms, and response to symptoms. Perception of symptoms refers to the participants' rating of the presence of symptoms and is obtained in two ways. First, a day-by-day rating is obtained from the 90-day diary. In addition, a retrospective symptom rating is obtained from the telephone interview conducted after the diary is completed. The items included in the health diary were generated from several sources (Halbreich, Endicott, Schach, & Nee, 1982; Moos, 1968, 1969).

Symptom evaluation refers to the subjective interpretation of symptoms, including the women's ratings of symptom severity, explanatory models for the causes of their symptoms, effects of symptoms on daily living, treatability of symptoms, attitudes toward menstruation, and perception of themselves as ill or well. Severity level is measured in the daily health diary. Effects on daily living, treatability, explanatory models, and perception of illness status are all included in the telephone interview. Menstrual attitudes are measured in the initial interview using the Menstrual Attitudes Scale (Brooks-Gunn & Ruble, 1980).

Response to symptoms includes actions taken, such as use of home remedies or health services, restriction of activity, and so on. Response is recorded on the daily health diary.

Socialization refers to the outcomes of social influences and includes both general socialization as a woman and socialization specific to menstruation. Indicators of general socialization as a woman include the Attitudes Toward Women Scale and Bem's scale to measure sex typing (see Spence & Helmreich, 1978). Socialization regarding menstruation is measured by women's recollections of menstruation (Brooks-Gunn & Ruble, 1980) and menstrual symptom expectancies (Paige, 1973). These items were included in the interview. Other indicators of socialization include education, political orientation, religion, family background, and ethnicity.

Social context refers to several dimensions of the woman's social environment. In particular, the dimensions of stress and support are considered. Norbeck's (1984) measure of stressful life events, a measure of the demands related to women's roles and their economic status, were included in the interview. Daily hassles were recorded for each day in the diary. A second dimension of the social environment is social support. Both the supportive and conflicted networks are measured using Barrerra's (1981) work.

Health practices are measured in the interview using indicators of exercise, diet, sleep and eating habits, alcohol use, and smoking. For a subsample of women with various symptom configurations, nutrient intake pattern is analyzed from eight days of food diary data—four from the follicular and four from the luteal phase. Exercise is recorded daily in the diary.

Reproductive health history is assessed in the interview and includes indicators of menstrual cycle characteristics, pregnancy history, contraceptive use, sterilization history, menarcheal experiences, postpartum depression, and other problems related to reproduction. Health status is also assessed in the interview, and includes the variables of depression, well-being, hospitalization in the last year, and therapy in the last year. In addition, a measure of the meaning of health is included in the telephone interview.

MODELING

Time and Its Measurement. The basic approach necessary to adequately develop a holistic understanding of menstrual cycle phenomena is multidimensional and dynamic. The approximately monthly pattern of the menstrual cycle itself indicates the dynamic character of this area. To look at a single point in time may reveal a striking pattern; but, as with a kaleidoscope, it is only one pattern of many that occurs with changes in the menstrual cycle. The time of studying the multiple dimensions, then, affects the patterns observed between the elements of the model.

The impact of time can perhaps be seen best in an example from physiological studies (Haskett, Steiner, & Carroll, 1984; Haskett, Steiner, Osmun, & Carroll, 1980). In recent years numerous cycle lengths have been identified, from very short ones lasting only seconds to others lasting a year. If only a single measurement is made or if a series of measurements is not of appropriate length, misleading information may be obtained. No single time can be considered representative of the status of the system of interest.

Cortisol nicely demonstrates the importance of time in making measurements. It has a circadian rhythm, with a peak in the early morning (usually just after the sleep period) and with minimum levels in the early evening. However, these levels are also influenced by the pulsatile pattern of secretion of cortisol. Thus, if a sample drawn in the evening were to coincide with a cortisol pulse, the level measured could exceed the ranges normally observed in the morning. Similarly, a single morning sample could have a value appropriate for the evening. Therefore, it is necessary to draw samples over enough time to ensure obtaining valid levels from both peaks and troughs, and to characterize the pattern of cortisol production adequately. Considering both the circadian characteristics and the pulsatile secretion pattern of cortisol, a twofold data collection scheme should be employed: first, measures across minutes should be made because of the pulsatile pattern; second, to identify the 24-hour rhythm, sampling must be done over the longer period as well.

Unlike cortisol, in which the sampling interval is measured in minutes and only over several days, gonadal hormone levels in the menstrual cycle have a period of interest that is several weeks long, and sampling must be spread over that time period. The sample must also be frequent enough to capture critical time points in the pattern of this hormone. Daily sampling could suffice at intervals of ovulation and in the premenstrual week, if these are the time periods of interest. Shorter time intervals would be needed to study daily variations. There is also some evidence of seasonal variation in the pattern of hormones and in the reported symptomatology every two to three cycles. This may reflect a seasonal as well as monthly rhythm. We may need, therefore, to apply time series analytic techniques to adjust our estimates seasonally. This seasonal variation also indicates the need to include measurements across several menstrual cycles. These hormone patterns do not exist in isolation, but they affect and are affected by other patterns and need to be studied in the context of those other patterns.

In sum, this example of cortisol and gonadal hormone illustrates the importance of adequately capturing time-related aspects and factors. They illustrate an important consideration for research on women's health.

Intraindividual Analysis. Analysis of data obtained serially begins appropriately at the level of the individual subject. Plotting individual data may allow investigators to study different patterns of phenomena across subjects that would have been masked if the data were only summarized as group data. For instance, some women have low symptom severity at all times of the menstrual cycle. Others have a pattern of increasing symptom severity, from low levels early in the menstrual cycle to higher levels in the premenstrual phase. The low-to-high pattern is the one most commonly reported in the literature; interestingly, however, it is the least commonly observed pattern in our sample. Instead, our approach to data analysis allowed us to detect both patterns characterized by either high or low symptom levels maintained across the entire menstrual cycle, and patterns that began with high symptom severity increasing to even higher symptom severity levels in the premenstrual week. These findings indeed justify the need for intraindividual analysis in our research project and highlight the need to consider this type of analysis more generally in women's health research.

The need for intraindividual analysis in women's health research is also evident in the area of emotions. The dynamic component in the emotional dimension requires the consideration of both trait and state characteristics. Traits are held to be relatively stable and characteristic of the individual regardless of the current situation. In contrast, state characteristics are held to vary in considerable degree across time and to reflect the current situation that the person is experiencing. One way of trying to determine more accurately if the reported emotional dimension is a state versus a trait is to repeat the measures across different situations to observe if the subject consistently reports similar emotional dimensions. In menstrual cycle research, one of the most consistently reported factors of premenstrual syndrome is negative affect. The question becomes, "Do the women manifest negative affect in relation to the menstrual cycle, or are they women who have negative affect at all times?" In the diary records, some women report high negative affect across all phases of the menstrual cycle with relatively higher levels at one phase. In contrast, other women report only low or minimal symptoms with increasing negative affect solely during the premenstrual phase. Only by having the daily record of these symptoms across several menstrual cycles is it possible to distinguish between these two groups. If a single measurement had been made of negative affect symptoms at the premenstrual phase, all women would have appeared to have essentially the same negative affect.

Cultural and Social Dynamics. In addition to the conventional approach of analyzing data across subjects and the need to complement this with intraindividual analyses, it is imperative to analyze women's health research data within a larger context of cultural and social dynamics. Indeed, the symptoms that are perceived as worthy of reporting vary from person to person and are shaped by the individual's culture or world view, previous experiences with similar conditions, and extent of disruption caused by the symptom. When women are asked to respond to a list of symptoms, their answers may vary because of how they notice and cognitively organize their symptoms. In menstrual research, for instance, it is important to find out whether women classify menstrual symptoms as a normal part of "being a woman" or as an illness.

Current stressful environmental elements constitute a dynamic influence on the perception of symptoms, and the culture of origin provides the overarching background for the individual's perceptions. In women's health research it may be helpful to consider the following: daily hassles, contemporary trends, changing economic opportunities, and political climate. These all represent ongoing influences and conditions in which the subject is immersed and which can be considered as a source of variation or trend in the pattern of responses observed.

To study the culture of origin, a straightforward single time of measurement should be adequate, as it is unlikely that major shifts in the underlying cultural norms and taboos, in which the subject has been raised, will occur rapidly. Less easy is the identification of the culture of origin. In our current study, we took the fairly standard approach of identifying different cultural groups on the basis of the country of origin of ancestors and of asking subjects to which ethnic group they belonged. We were surprised when subjects said they did not know what country most of their family came from, but emphasized that they came from, say, "Mississippi" or "the Mid-West." This type of response suggests that in the consideration of culture of origin, it is important to think through the notion of cultural group or subgroup. Ethnographic work can serve as a useful resource for identifying such nontraditional cultural groups and subgroups and for clarifying the sociocultural content to be investigated.

Conclusion

In this chapter we linked issues in women's health and nursing with an ongoing research project. Women's health research is indeed at a point at which the mere enumeration of issues and problems would be uninformative. In our research we have confronted some of these issues, and an "operational" discussion of them on the basis of actual research was considered more advantageous. More generally, in our work we have tried to encompass within our measures and analyses some of the dynamism and holism that is women's health. We believe that through such approaches nursing science can match the richness of its conceptual frameworks with equally rich measurement and analysis.

REFERENCES

Barnard, K. (1980). Knowledge for practice: Directions for the future. *Nursing Research, 26*, 113–120.

Barrera, M. (1981). Social support in the adjustment of pregnant adolescents: Assessment issues. In B. Gottlieb (Ed.), *Social networks and social support* (pp. 69–96). Beverly Hills: Sage.

Brooks-Gunn, J., & Ruble, D. (1980). The menstrual attitude questionnaire. *Psychosomatic Medicine, 42*, 503–512.

Chrisman, N., & Kleinman, A. (1983). Popular health care, social networks, and cultural meanings: The orientation of medical anthropology. In D. Mechanic (Ed.), *Handbook of health care and health professions* (pp. 569–590). New York: Free Press.

Halbreich, U., Endicott, J., Schach, S., & Nee, J. (1982). The diversity of premenstrual changes as reflected in the premenstrual assessment form. *Acta Psychiatrica Scandinavica, 62*, 177–180.

Haskett, R., Steiner, M., & Carroll, B. (1984). A psychoendocrine study of premenstrual tension syndrome: A model for endogenous depression? *Journal of Affective Disorders, 6*, 191–199.

Haskett, R., Steiner, M., Osmun, J., & Carroll, B. (1980). Severe premenstrual tension: Delineation of the syndrome. *Biological Psychiatry, 15*, 121–139.

McBride, A., & McBride, W. (1981). Theoretical underpinnings of women's health. *Women and Health, 6*, 37–55.

Moos, R. H. (1968). The development of a menstrual distress questionnaire. *Psychosomatic Medicine, 30*, 853–867.

Moos, R. H. (1969). Typology of menstrual cycle symptoms. *American Journal of Obstetrics and Gynecology, 103,* 390–402.

Norbeck, J. (1984). Modification of life event questionnaires for use with female respondents. *Research in Nursing and Health, 7,* 61–71.

Paige, K. (1973). Women learn to sing the menstrual blues. *Psychology Today, 7,* 41–46.

Spence, J., Helmreich, R. (1978). *Masculinity and femininity: Their psychological dimensions, correlates, and antecedents.* Austin: University of Texas Press.

Woods, N. (1988). Women's health: A review of the last five years. *Annual Review of Nursing Research, 6,* 209–236.

Comment

On the Future of Women's and Reproductive Health Research

SUSAN KUTZNER, Ph.D., R.N.

It is only recently that a research movement focused on women and their health issues has emerged. Yet, notwithstanding its young history, it is important to speculate about the future of this field and, as much as possible, to formulate directives for this future. Departing from the previous chapter by Lentz and Woods, some general design and analysis issues are raised that are relevant to future scientific efforts.

As a general comment, the term women's health was useful to place a specific emphasis on women during the 1960s and 1970s. The more appropriate term for this and the following decade might be reproductive health to denote health issues from psychological, physiological, social, and other perspectives that include men as well as women. Perhaps we are being unnecessarily sexist in the greater emphasis on women.

The preceding chapter offers a thorough perspective on research on women's health. A number of important issues are raised, and suggestions for the future are made. The actual research cited offers a helpful example and underscores in an operational mode the main points of the chapter. A few extensions and additions might be helpful.

If one looks at the research in the field of women's health from approximately 1970 to the present, a pattern becomes apparent.

The vast majority of the studies are within the client domain, utilizing nonnursing frameworks to structure investigations. Quite a few of these studies utilize unidimensional research designs and limited quantitative methods and procedures. Only a few studies are focused on the practice domain, and even fewer studies fall in the domain of client–nurse interaction. It is timely and pertinent to change this pattern into one that encompasses studies on dynamic interactional phenomena, perhaps within a developmental–maturational framework. Research in the field might also benefit from an interactional theoretical model. Lentz and Woods should be supported in their case for longitudinal designs, for these might capture most accurately cyclical or recurrent physiological and psychological themes.

The past and current emphasis on nonexperimental studies will, in the long run, not yield the depth of knowledge that is clinically and socially mandated. Nonexperimental research merely establishes that relationships exist among variables. However, without manipulation of putative causes, it is difficult to make causal inferences. Experimental or quasi-experimental designs should be promoted instead in the future.

A large proportion of the research since 1970 utilizes self-report questionnaires, diaries, or interviews. Most often only one method is chosen to measure a particular variable, and multi-method studies are indeed remarkably absent. Studies with multiple measurement approaches, particularly with data collection methods that assure noninteraction of measures, would be more powerful. Given the relationships that exist between physiological and psychological variables, an integrated and comprehensive psychophysiological perspective must be advocated.

In summary, in addition to the recommendations made in the preceding chapter, the following foci should be encouraged within women's *and* reproductive health research: (1) investigations, preferably within a programmatic context, in the domains of client and client–nurse interaction; (2) multimethod approaches with a comprehensive psychophysiological focus, used within research paradigms that permit the inference of casuality; and (3) a stronger emphasis on and sophistication of statistical methodology.

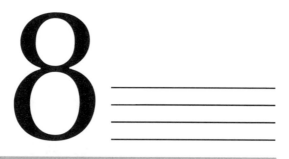

8

A Statistical Evaluation of the Psychiatric Nursing Research Literature

SUSAN L. JONES, Ph.D., F.A.A.N.
PAUL K. JONES, Ph.D.

Statistics is the science whereby inferences are made about specific random phenomena on the basis of sample material. The field of statistics can be subdivided into two main areas: mathematical and applied statistics. Mathematical statistics is concerned with the development of new methods of statistical inference. Applied statistics, which is our concern here, is the application of the methods of mathematical statistics to specific subject areas such as economics, psychology, public health, nursing, and so on. Biostatistics is the branch of applied statistics concerned with the application of statistical methods to nursing, medical, and biological problems (Rosner, 1982).

The focus of this chapter is on examining the appropriateness of use and sophistication level of statistical methods in psychiatric nursing research. The first task of such an examination is to clarify conceptually the unit of analysis, that is, "research in psychiatric nursing." Here we must distinguish psychiatric *nursing* from the other mental health disciplines; we must distinguish *psychiatric* nursing from the other clinical nursing specialties; and we must *identify* what is meant by *research*.

Exactly when clinical interventions with psychiatric patients, or observations of psychological behavior, or measurement of psychological attitudes fall within the realm of psychiatric nursing is at times difficult to determine. It is not the purpose of this chapter to discuss the issue of nursing versus nonnursing observations or interventions. However, it is essential that criteria be established for identification of nursing research studies. One such criterion is that only nursing journals were used as the source for studies in the following analysis. Obviously, therefore, this analysis is not exhaustive. Many psychiatric nurses have published nursing research articles in other than nursing journals. It is our belief, however, that articles published in nursing journals adequately represent the current integration and use of statistics in psychiatric nursing.

It is also difficult at times to distinguish a psychiatric nursing study from a study that would be classified as nursing-based, but in an area other than psychiatric nursing. The following review includes only articles that involve psychiatric nursing in a more traditional sense. Thus, articles that addressed psychosocial aspects of nursing care are omitted.

There is no doubt that psychiatric liaison nursing has become more and more prominent in recent years within the field of psychiatric nursing. Indeed, several studies that involve psychiatric liaison nursing are included in this review. However, unless a study was identified as specifically involving psychiatric liaison nursing in some manner, studies that examined psychosocial aspects of nonpsychiatric patients were not included here.

The final distinction involves the question of when collection of empirical data constitutes a study. Only formal studies are included here. Reports on clinical vignettes, hypothetical studies that could be designed, case studies, and application of theoretical concepts to clinical practice are not included. Omission of these nonformal studies is particularly important, since this review examines statistical techniques used; the nonformal studies, such as a case study, frequently utilize no statistical analysis.

Method and Materials

An analysis of the adequacy of *theory development* within psychiatric nursing has been conducted (O'Toole, 1981). However, a statistical evaluation of psychiatric nursing research has not been done to date, although statistical evaluations and criteria for adequacy have been outlined for research in social science and medicine. We thus chose to use this statistical literature as a guideline to assure that our evaluation criteria and approach would be consistent with statistical evaluations done previously. Using these statistical criteria (Fleiss, Tytun, & Ury, 1980; Gehan, 1980; Lachan, 1982; Mosteller, 1981; O'Fallon, Dubey, Salsburg, Edmonson, Soffer, & Colton, 1978; Shor & Karten, 1966; Thibodeau, 1980; Virgo, 1977) as well as established criteria from critique outlines in standard statistical and research methodology texts (Keppel, 1973; Kerlinger, 1973; Kirk, 1982; Polit & Hungler, 1983), we established our criteria for evaluation of each article reported here.

A prerequisite to a good statistical analysis is a good study design (Huck, Cormier, & Bounds, 1974). Statistical procedures must be appropriate for the study design. The number of variables and/or number of groups must be appropriate in relation to the sample size. Clear conceptual and operational definitions are necessary to measure variables adequately. And most important, there must be a clear statement of the problem to guide the overall method of study.

In sum, statistical procedures cannot be evaluated apart from other methodological components of a study. In the following critique, therefore, we address several design aspects of reported research in addition to the statistical methods outlined in the studies.

Each article was subjected to an intensive critical reading independently by each author. The article was then discussed and evaluated according to specified methodological and statistical criteria. We did not try to assess the relative merits of the research question itself, that is, whether the question should be addressed in the first place. Rather, we confined our critique to evaluation of the methodology and statistical procedures used. Each article was classified by journal type; year of publication; author characteristics; number and type of references; conceptual clarity; kind of study or design; numbers of subjects, variables, and groups; type of statistical procedures used; kinds of statistics reported; and whether differences in groups were found and, if so, what kind.

Findings

CHARACTERISTICS OF AUTHORS AND JOURNALS

For this analysis, we reviewed 24 journals between the years 1970 and 1985. Of these journals, 153 psychiatric nursing articles were found in 15 journals. Nine journals contained no psychiatric nursing articles. Although the journal survey may have inadvertently failed to locate certain articles, the survey is essentially a population survey rather than a sampling of articles. Accordingly, no inferential statistical procedures were used to compare percentages or means in the following report.

Table 8–1 presents the percent of articles classified by nursing journal type. Four classifications were used: journals with research articles only; journals with theoretical, clinical, and research articles; psychiatric clinical journals; and nonpsychiatric clinical journals. The preponderant journal group consisted of psychiatric clinical journals, with 51% of the journal articles. The next most frequent journal type was research, with 32%.

Table 8–2 shows a comparison of author characteristics by journal classification. On the average, there were 1.9 authors per article, a finding that was constant across journal classifications. Forty-five percent of authors had doctorates as their highest degree, 42% had master's degrees, and 10% had baccalaureates. Over two thirds (79%) were nurses, with the highest percent

TABLE 8–1. PERCENTAGE OF ARTICLES CLASSIFIED
BY NURSING JOURNAL

Journal	Number of Articles	Percent
Research	(49)	(32)
International Journal of Nursing Studies	9	6
Nursing Research	30	20
Research in Nursing and Health	5	3
Western Journal of Nursing Research	5	3
Theoretical–Clinical–Research	(13)	(8)
Advances in Nursing Science	2	1
Image	1	below 1
Journal of Advanced Nursing	10	6
Clinical, Psychiatric	(78)	(51)
Issues in Mental Health Nursing	26	17
Journal of Psychosocial Nursing	46	30
Perspectives in Psychiatric Care	6	4
Clinical, Nonpsychiatric	(13)	(8)
Heart and Lung	9	6
Journal of Gerontological Nursing	1	below 1
Journal of Obstetrics and Gynecological Nursing	1	below 1
Maternal Child Nursing	1	below 1
Public Health Nursing	1	below 1
Total	153	100%

TABLE 8–2. COMPARISON OF AUTHOR CHARACTERISTICS
BY JOURNAL CLASSIFICATION

Characteristic	Research, $N = 49$	Theoretical, Clinical, Research, $N = 13$	Clinical, Psychiatric, $N = 78$	Clinical, Nonpsychiatric, $N = 13$	Total, $N = 153$
Mean number of authors per article	1.8	1.8	1.8	2.3	1.9
Percent of Authors					
With doctorates	47	38	43	57	45
With master's	40	50	46	20	42
With baccalaureates	14	12	8	7	10
Who are nurses	78	50	72	43	69
Who are M.D.s	4	0	8	23	7
Who conducted study in fulfillment of academic degree	18	15	38	31	29
Who had financial support for study	26	0	14	15	19
Percent of First Authors					
Who are nurses	90	62	86	69	84
Who are nurses with doctorates	47	8	31	8	32
Who are nurses with master's	35	31	47	31	40
Who are M.D.s	0	0	3	0	1

TABLE 8–3. COMPARISON OF CHARACTERISTICS BY YEAR OF PUBLICATION

Characteristic	1970–74, N = 20	1975–79, N = 46	1980–85, N = 87	Total, N = 153
Mean number of authors/article	1.9	1.9	1.8	1.9
Percent of Authors				
With doctorates	50	40	48	45
With master's	28	44	45	42
With baccalaureates	16	16	4	10
Who are nurses	63	61	75	69
Who are M.D.s	15	11	3	7
Who conducted study in fulfillment of academic degree	10	24	37	29
Who had financial support for study	10	28	16	19
Percent of First Authors				
Who are nurses	85	83	84	84
Who are nurses with doctorates	25	28	36	32
Who are nurses with master's	40	37	42	40
Who are M.D.s	10	0	0	1

of nurses (78%) represented in research journals. Clinical nonpsychiatric journals constituted the journal type in which the fewest nurses (43%) were represented. Only 7% of the authors were physicians, and most of the articles in which physicians were authors were in clinical psychiatric and clinical nonpsychiatric journals. Nearly one third (29%) of the studies were conducted in fulfillment of the requirements of an academic degree. About one fifth (19%) of the studies were conducted with some type of financial support, which included local, state, or federal funding.

Examination of first authors indicated that 84% were nurses, with the higher percentages being represented in research journals (90%) and clinical psychiatric journals (86%). Less than one third (32%) of first authors were nurses with doctorates, and 40% were nurses with a master's degree as the highest degree. Only 1% of first authors were physicians.

Table 8–3 presents a comparison of author characteristics by year of publication. The right-most column in this table is identical to that in Table 8–2. Other columns show changes in author characteristics by five-year intervals. The mean number of authors did not change. Although the percentage of authors with doctorates remained quite stable (about 40% to 50%), the percentage of authors with master's degrees increased from 28% to 45% in the 16-year span. Conversely, the percentage of authors with at most a baccalaureate degree declined from 16% to 4%. The percentage of nurse authors increased from 63% to 75%, whereas the percentage of physician authors declined from 15% to 3%. There was an increase in the percentage

TABLE 8–4. MEAN AND RANGE OF NUMBERS OF REFERENCES

Characteristic	Research, N = 49	Theoretical, Clinical, Research, N = 13	Clinical, Psychiatric, N = 78	Clinical, Nonpsychiatric, N = 13	Total, N = 153
Mean number of references	18 (4-57)	12 (4-48)	17 (0-53)	18 (2-27)	17 (0-57)
Mean number of statistical references	0.3 (0-2)	0.0 (0-0)	0.2 (0-3)	0.3 (0-2)	0.2 (0-3)

of studies conducted in fulfillment of degree requirements (10% to 37%), whereas the percentage of studies receiving financial support showed no systematic change over time.

Looking at changes over time in the characteristics of first authors showed that the percentage of first authors who are nurses remained high (83% to 85%) over the 16-year span. The percentage of doctorally prepared first authors increased from 25% to 36%, and the percentage of nurses with a master's degree remained relatively constant. In the time period of 1970–1974, 10% of first authors were physicians; subsequently, no physicians were first authors.

The mean and range of number of references in each journal classification is presented in Table 8–4. The mean number of references is 17, with a range of 0 to 57. Few statistical references are presented in the journals (0.2 average, with a range of 0 to 3).

METHODOLOGICAL CHARACTERISTICS OF STUDIES

Table 8–5 shows that the most common kind of study conducted was cross-sectional (79%). No differences were apparent by journal classification. The next most frequent type of study was longitudinal (12%).

TABLE 8–5. KIND OF STUDY BY NURSING JOURNAL CLASSIFICATION

Characteristic	Research, N = 49	Theoretical, Clinical Research, N = 13	Clinical, Psychiatric, N = 78	Clinical, Nonpsychiatric, N = 13	Total, N = 153
Longitudinal	8%	38%	9%	23%	72%
Cross-sectional	78%	62%	85%	77%	19%
Record review	4%	0%	4%	0%	3%
Methodological study	8%	0%	1%	0%	4%
Historical study	0%	0%	1%	0%	1%
Case history	2%	0%	0%	0%	1%
Total	100%	100%	100%	100%	100%

TABLE 8–6. TYPE OF DESIGN BY NURSING JOURNAL CLASSIFICATION

Design	Research, N = 49	Theoretical, Clinical, Research, N = 13	Clinical, Psychiatric, N = 78	Clinical, Nonpsychiatric, N = 13	Total, N = 153
Descriptive	74%	69%	64%	92%	72%
Quasi-experimental	12%	31%	18%	8%	16%
Experimental (classical)	6%	0%	9%	0%	7%
Ethnographic	8%	0%	9%	0%	5%
Total	100%	100%	100%	100%	100%

Table 8–6 presents the type of study design by nursing journal classification. Descriptive studies were the most frequent (72%). If we combine the experimental and quasi-experimental, these studies accounted for nearly one fourth (23%) of the sample.

The number of subjects, variables, and groups by journal classification is presented in Table 8–7. Six percent of the studies were methodological or ethnographic and did not have subjects. We classified those studies that had subjects into three groups: 1–25, 26–75, and over 75 subjects. Roughly one third of the sample fell within each group.

In our analysis, we distinguished between the number of variables studied and the number of groups studied. A variable here represents a

TABLE 8–7. NUMBER OF SUBJECTS, VARIABLES, AND GROUPS BY JOURNAL CLASSIFICATION

Characteristic	Research, N = 49	Theoretical, Clinical, Research, N = 13	Clinical, Psychiatric, N = 78	Clinical, Nonpsychiatric, N = 13	Total, N = 153
Number of Subjects					
None	8%	0%	8%	0%	6%
1-25	22%	23%	28%	54%	28%
26-75	33%	23%	37%	46%	36%
over 75	37%	54%	27%	0%	30%
Total	100%	100%	100%	100%	100%
Number of Variables					
1	59%	46%	49%	46%	52%
2	18%	46%	28%	54%	29%
3 or more	23%	8%	23%	0%	19%
Total	100%	100%	100%	100%	100%
Number of Groups					
1	45%	15%	49%	69%	46%
2	39%	46%	38%	31%	39%
3 or more	16%	39%	13%	0%	15%
Total	100%	100%	100%	100%	100%

TABLE 8–8. CONCEPTUAL CLARITY BY JOURNAL CLASSIFICATION

Characteristic	Research, $N = 49$	Theoretical, Clinical, Research, $N = 13$	Clinical, Psychiatric, $N = 78$	Clinical, Nonpsychiatric, $N = 13$	Total, $N = 153$
Theoretical/ Conceptual Framework	46%	8%	31%	15%	33%
Clarity of Statement of Problem					
Very clear	74%	38%	63%	77%	65%
Less clear	26%	62%	37%	23%	35%
Total	100%	100%	100%	100%	100%
Adequacy of Definitions					
Conceptual & operational	56%	28%	46%	92%	51%
Conceptual only	16%	0%	6%	0%	8%
Operational only	24%	77%	28%	8%	29%
None	4%	0%	20%	0%	12%
Total	100%	100%	100%	100%	100%
Sample Described Statistically					
Yes	59%	38%	40%	69%	49%
Vague	4%	0%	4%	0%	3%
No	35%	62%	55%	31%	47%
Not applicable	2%	0%	1%	0%	1%
Total	100%	100%	100%	100%	100%

major "study" variable, that is, the variable was outlined in the study purpose, study question, or hypothesis. Subjects may additionally be divided into groups, where the groups do not include study variables.

The purpose of distinguishing between variables and groups was to permit classification of studies according to the statistical tests employed in the analysis of data. For example, a t-test could be conducted on a single variable (e.g., depression) for two groups (e.g., males and females). Alternatively, a correlation could be computed for health status and depression (two variables) within a single group.

Over half of the studies (52%) involved analysis of a single variable, nearly one third (29%) involved two variables, and one fifth (19%) had three or more variables. These percentages are relatively constant across journal type. Nearly half of the studies (46%) contained only one group, 39% contained two groups, and only 15% involved three or more groups.

CONCEPTUAL CLARITY

Table 8–8 presents evaluations of the conceptual clarity of articles by journal classification. Whether an article contained a theoretical framework

TABLE 8–9. TYPE OF STATISTICAL PROCEDURES USED
BY JOURNAL CLASSIFICATION

Characteristic	Research, N = 49	Theoretical, Clinical, Research, N = 13	Clinical, Psychiatric, N = 78	Clinical, Nonpsychiatric, N = 13	Total, N = 153
Statistical Procedures Used					
Descriptive	35%	39%	51%	31%	43%
Descriptive + parametric inferential	43%	31%	23%	23%	30%
Descriptive + nonparametric inferential	12%	15%	20%	23%	18%
Descriptive + combination	8%	15%	3%	15%	6%
Does not say	2%	0%	3%	8%	3%
Total	100%	100%	100%	100%	100%
Type of Analysis					
Univariate	51%	31%	52%	39%	49%
Bivariate	33%	38%	42%	46%	39%
Multivariate	16%	31%	6%	15%	12%
Total	100%	100%	100%	100%	100%

was determined according to whether or not the article contained a broad conceptual basis as a backdrop within which to discuss the nature of the question and the study results. Using this criterion, one third of the articles (33%) involved a theoretical framework.

Approximately two thirds (65%) of the studies were judged to have a very clear statement of the problem. A study was judged to have a less clear statement of the problem when the exact purpose of the study was not stated or the study variables were not outlined in the problem statement. The most frequent mistake in outlining the problem was stating that the purpose of the study was to show the relationship between two variables, when in actuality there were three variables in the study design.

About half (51%) of the articles provided adequate definitions at both the conceptual and operational level. It was more common to provide an adequate operational definition than an adequate conceptual definition. The operational definitions were more apt to be included, since the article was likely to contain a description of the instrument used. About half (49%) of the studies included a statistical description of the sample.

STATISTICAL PROCEDURES USED

The types of statistical procedures used by journal classification are presented in Table 8–9. The most frequent type of procedure was descriptive (43%). However, various combinations of inferential statistical procedures accounted for over half (54%) of the studies. Of those, the most common form was descriptive plus parametric statistics (30%).

Each analysis was classified as univariate (one variable), bivariate (two

**TABLE 8–10. STATISTICAL CHARACTERISTICS OF ARTICLE
BY SAMPLE SIZE**

| | Sample Size Range | | | |
Characteristic	1–25, N = 43	26–75, N = 54	Over 75, N = 46	Total N = 153
Kind of Statistics Reported				
Descriptive only	56%	30%	41%	43%
Descriptive + parametric inferential	23%	39%	30%	30%
Descriptive + nonparametric inferential	14%	19%	20%	18%
Descriptive + combination	7%	7%	7%	6%
Does not say	0%	5%	2%	3%
Total	100%	100%	100%	100%
Number of Groups				
1	70%	44%	36%	46%
2	26%	41%	46%	39%
3 or more	4%	15%	18%	15%
Total	100%	100%	100%	100%
Number of Variables in Analysis				
1 (univariate)	58%	39%	46%	49%
2 (bivariate)	33%	50%	37%	39%
3 or more (multivariate)	9%	11%	17%	12%
Total	100%	100%	100%	100%

Note: A total of 10 studies did not have any statistical characteristics.

variables), or multivariate (three or more variables). Half (49%) of the analyses were univariate; 39% were bivariate; and only 12% were multivariate.

STATISTICAL PROCEDURES, NUMBERS OF GROUPS, AND VARIABLES

Table 8–10 presents the type of statistics used, the number of groups, and the number of variables in the analysis, by sample size—that is, the number of subjects specified in the journal article. The right-most column of this table corresponds to the right-most column of Table 8–9. With increasing sample size, there tended to be a decrease in the percentage of articles employing descriptive statistics only (56% to 30%), although the trend was not consistent. Conversely, there tended to be an increase in the percentage employing some parametric inference (23% to 39%), although again the trend was not consistent. In general, the larger the sample size of the article, the larger was the observed percentage of articles identifying three or more groups of subjects. That is, the percentage of articles identifying three or more groups increased (from 4% to 18%) as the number of subjects per article increased. The percentage of articles employing either bivariate or multivariate tests (range 42% to 61%) tended to increase with sample size in the article, although the trend was not consistent.

TABLE 8–11. PERCENT OF ARTICLES REPORTING TESTS ON MEANS BY SAMPLE SIZE

Characteristic	1–25, N = 43	26–75, N = 54	Over 75, N = 46	Total, N = 153
Student's t-test	7%	22%	17%	15%
Analysis of variance	9%	11%	9%	9%
Analysis of covariance	2%	0%	%	1%
Multiple regression	0%	2%	4%	2%
Discriminant analysis or nonparametric analysis	2%	2%	2%	2%
Correlation analysis	16%	13%	11%	13%
Combination	2%	6%	5%	5%
No inferential test used	62%	44%	50%	53%
Total	100%	100%	100%	100%

Note: A total of 10 studies did not have any statistical characteristics.

Table 8–11 shows the statistical procedures on means that are used by sample size within articles. The most common procedure involving comparison of means was found to consist of *not* performing an inferential test at all (53%). When an inferential procedure was used, it was most likely to be the student's *t*-test (15%) or correlation analysis (13%). No general pattern by type of statistical procedure was apparent across the different sample sizes of studies.

Table 8–12 presents a parallel analysis of statistical procedures for proportions by sample size within articles. Again, the most common procedure involving comparison of proportions was *not* to perform an inferential test at all (80%). When an inferential procedure on proportions was used, it was most likely to be the chi-square test (14%).

SAMPLE SIZE: THEORETICAL CONSIDERATIONS

An important consideration in the design of studies is the sample size. The power of an inferential statistical test is dependent upon the sample

TABLE 8–12. PERCENT OF ARTICLES REPORTING TESTS ON PROPORTIONS BY SAMPLING SIZE

Characteristic	1–25, N = 43	26–75, N = 54	Over 75, N = 46	Total, N = 153
Test on single proportion	2%	0%	0%	1%
Test for difference of two proportions	2%	0%	4%	2%
Chi-square	2%	18%	20%	14%
Sign test	0%	2%	0%	1%
Combination	2%	2%	2%	2%
No inferential test used	92%	78%	74%	80%
Total	100%	100%	100%	100%

Note: A total of 10 studies did not have any statistical characteristics.

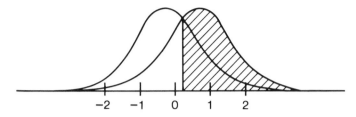

Situation A: Two-Group Comparison:
Normal Curve Displaced One Half Standard Deviation to the Right
(Substantial overlap in observations made for subjects in different groups)

	Required Sample Size Per Group at .05 Significance Level	
Power	**t-test**	**Chi-square**
.50	32	96
.80	64	194
.90	86	258
.95	106	318

Assuming ratio of difference of population means to SD is one half.
Assuming population proportions are 0.40 and 0.60.

Figure 8–1.

size, the number of groups in the analysis, the magnitude of population differences, and the analytic technique used. As was shown earlier, the total sample size for the studies falls roughly into thirds, with one third being 1 to 25, one third being 26 to 75, and one third being greater than 75 subjects. The magnitude of population differences varied from study to study, from very small to very great differences. The number of groups varied, but the most common comparisons involved either two or three groups.

The following section presents a description of two extreme situations requiring very different sample sizes. The purpose of this presentation is to permit evaluation of the reason inferential differences in groups were or were not detected. In an evaluation of use of statistical procedures it is important to determine whether differences (or lack thereof) were found because of a certain sample size, a certain number of groups being investigated, a certain magnitude of population differences, or the analytic procedure used.

Figure 8–1 (Situation A) describes an instance in which it is desired to compare two groups in which the individual observations overlap substantially. The depicted difference is assumed to be clinically important to the investigator. In Situation A it is assumed that the distributions of measurements on the study variable are described by two normal curves. The two curves have equal standard deviations but have means that differ by one half of the common standard deviation. Using standard statistical tables (Beyer, 1971), the number of subjects required to attain statistical powers of .50, .80, .90, and .95 were computed for the t-test. A two-tailed test with significance level of .05 was assumed.

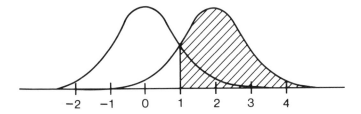

Situation B: Two-Group Comparison:
Normal Curve Displaced Two Standard Deviations to the Right
(Little overlap in observations made for subjects in different groups)

| | Required Sample Size per Group at .05 Significance Level | |
Power	t-test[*]	Chi-square[+]
.50	4	8
.80	6	14
.90	7	18
.95	8	22

[*]Assuming ratio of difference of population means to SD is 2.0.
[+]Assuming the population proportions are 0.16 and 0.84.

Figure 8–2.

Situation A was also used to compute the power of the chi-square test. It was assumed that the continuous normal variable was dichotomized in both groups and that the shaded area in Figure 8–1 represents the probabilities of observing a "positive response." In the left-hand curve the probability of a "positive response" is .40 and in the right hand curve it is .60. Using a standard table (Fleiss, 1982), the required sample sizes to attain powers of .50, .80, .90, and .95 were computed. The values for the chi-square test were larger than those for the t-test for equivalent power.

With either the t-test or chi-square test, the number of observations per group required to reach a power of .95 may exceed the resources of an investigator. Thus, if the magnitude of the differences between populations is small (i.e., Situation A), the investigator may be unable to assure sufficient power unless extremely large sample sizes are attained. The result is a Type II error, or failing to find a difference in the populations when a difference does indeed exist.

Figure 8–2 (Situation B) describes an instance in which it is desired to compare two groups in which the individual observations overlap much less. In this depiction the difference is assumed to be not only clinically important but also easy to find. Here it is assumed that two normal curves have the same standard deviation, but have means that differ by two standard deviations. Using standard statistical tables (Beyer, 1971), power was calculated for the t-test as in Figure 8–1. To compute power for the chi-square test the continuous normally distributed variable was dichotomized as indicated in Figure 8–2. The proportion in the shaded area is .16 for the left-hand curve and .84 for the right-hand curve. Using a standard table

TABLE 8–13. MEAN SAMPLE SIZE PER GROUP
BY SAMPLE SIZE RANGE AND NUMBER OF GROUPS*

Number of Groups	Sample Size Range		
	1–25	26–75	Over 75
1	13	40	191
	(30)[†]	(24)	(12)
2	8	24	89
	(11)	(22)	(21)
3	4	18	74
	(1)	(6)	(6)

*Excluding articles that studied more than three groups.
[†]The number of articles in each cell is in parentheses.

(Fleiss, 1982) the required sample sizes were obtained for the chi-square test to attain the same powers of .50, .80, .90, and .95. In general, the sample sizes for the chi-square test were again larger than those required for the *t*-test.

With either the *t*-test or chi-square test the number of observations per group to reach a power of .95 in Situation B is much less than in Situation A. That is, the sample sizes can be minimal to reach statistically significant differences in groups in Situation B.

SAMPLE SIZE: EMPIRICAL OBSERVATIONS

Table 8–13 depicts mean sample size per group by total sample size range and number of groups. Articles that studied more than three groups were omitted because there were very few of them and this obscured the comparison. Studies involving one group had a sample size averaging 13 in the sample size range of 1–25, 48 in the sample size range of 26–75, and 191 in the sample size range of over 75. Studies involving two groups had a sample size per group averaging 8, 24, and 89 in these respective ranges. Thus, a *t*-test comparing means of two groups would have inadequate power in Situation A except for the largest sample size range. The *t*-test would have adequate power in Situation B for all sample size ranges. The point at which a particular study falls between Situation A and Situation B is empirically determined and depends upon the magnitude of differences under study in the populations considered relative to the within-groups variability. The greater the difference between groups holding within-group variability constant, the more likely it is that the investigator will detect a difference.

Sample size per group in each sample range is lessened as the number of groups increases. Thus, the more groups that are studied, the greater the demand for substantial population differences to detect a difference using inferential statistical procedures. For example, with three groups the average sample size per group is 4 in the sample size range of 1–25; 18 in the sample size range of 26–75; and 74 in the sample size range of greater than 75.

TABLE 8–14. REPORT OF FINDINGS
IN TWO GROUP COMPARISONS BY SAMPLE SIZE

| Findings | Sample Size Range | | | |
	1–25, N = 11	26–75, N = 22	Over 75, N = 21	Total, N = 54
Did not test differences in groups	9%	27%	38%	28%
Descriptive difference not found	9%	0%	0%	2%
Inferential differences not found	27%	14%	5%	13%
Reported differences descriptively	9%	0%	14%	7%
Reported differences inferentially	46%	59%	43%	50%
Total	100%	100%	100%	100%

Table 8–14 summarizes the type of finding in two group comparisons by sample size range. In the total sample involving two group comparisons, 50% reported the detection of differences using inferential statistics. Surprisingly, the percentage reporting the detection of such differences does not correspond to sample size ranges. That is, regardless of the study sample size, approximately one half (range 43% to 59%) of the studies reported detection of differences inferentially.

PREDICTING THE DETECTION OF INFERENTIAL DIFFERENCES IN GROUPS

The question now becomes one of why did some studies find differences inferentially while others did not, and how can it be explained that inferential differences were not related to sample size? To answer this question, we again examined those studies that detected inferential differences and those that did not.

Our first hypothesis was that use of a standardized instrument versus one constructed by the author would allow for greater reliability and sensitivity of measurement and could partially explain why some researchers found inferential differences and others did not. Of those investigators who used standardized instruments, 54% detected differences inferentially, and of those who did not use standardized instruments, only 24% detected such differences.

Our second hypothesis was that those investigators testing the same subjects at more than one time point would detect differences inferentially, since a repeated-measures design would be more efficient. This hypothesis was not supported, because, of the studies using a repeated-measures design, 42% detected inferential differences versus 37% of those not using a repeated-measures design.

Our third hypothesis was that Situation B (minimal overlap between groups compared) occurred more frequently for those studies in which inferential differences were found. Thus, in Situation B a very small sample size is required to detect differences in the two groups. An examination of those articles that detected inferential differences and those that did not supported this hypothesis, although a systematic comparison was not always possible because the unit of analysis of studies differed. We present some examples studied in the articles to highlight what we consider to be a major reason that some investigators detected inferential differences and others did not.

Differences Found. Looking first at those articles in which investigators detected differences, we clinically and intuitively found minimal overlap between groups (Situation B). For example, in one study (DiVasto, 1985) involving 118 subjects and two groups, the phenomena of rape was studied, comparing rape victims with a group of female undergraduate nursing students. Inferential differences were found on the dependent variables, which included sleep disorders, appetite problems, phobias and fears, self-esteem, and so on. Our hypothesis is that the two groups—rape victims and control subjects—represented two distinctly different groups with minimal overlap on the variables studied in the first place.

A second example of a study in which inferential differences were found and in which we hypothesize minimal overlap between groups (Situation B) involves a descriptive study of the Mount St. Helens disaster (Murphy, 1984). Five levels of the independent variable of loss were outlined with a total sample size of 155. Loss was operationally defined in terms of degree of loss of a relative or friend (presumed dead or confirmed dead) and/or loss of property (permanent residence or leisure residence). A control group of individuals who had no loss from the disaster but who were matched on demographic variables was included as well. Subjects per group ranged from 15 to 39. The dependent variables studied were stress and health. Findings showed differences in groups on the different dependent variables. Again, our hypothesis is that the two groups compared represented two groups with minimal overlap on the variables studied.

Differences Not Found. Looking at those articles that used inferential statistics but that did *not* detect differences, we intuitively and clinically hypothesize overlaps between groups to be closer to Situation A, that is, substantial overlap between groups. For example, in one study (Gibson, 1980) involving 61 male alcoholic patients, the phenomena of self-esteem and the satisfaction with that self-esteem were studied as a dependent variable. The independent variable was a reminiscence group whereby the experimental group received a reminiscence group intervention and the control group did not. The impact of the reminiscence group on self-esteem was examined with no differences being found between groups. Our hypothesis is that the two groups being compared (i.e., experimental and

	Sample Size Range			
Findings	1–25, N = 2	26–75, N = 8	Over 75, N = 13	Total, N = 23
Did not test differences in groups	0%	25%	15%	17%
Descriptive differences not found	0%	0%	8%	4%
Inferential differences not found	0%	12%	0%	4%
Reported differences descriptively	0%	12%	8%	9%
Reported differences inferentially	100%	50%	69%	66%
Total	100%	100%	100%	100%

TABLE 8–15. REPORT OF FINDINGS IN GROUP COMPARISONS INVOLVING AT LEAST THREE GROUPS BY SAMPLE SIZE

control group alcoholic patients) overlap substantially on the dependent variables of interest.

A second example of a study in which no inferential differences were found was a study examining the potential relationship between previous elective abortions and postpartum depressive reactions (Devore, 1979). This study involved 48 primiparous women, 25 of whom had had one abortion previously. No significant differences in depression between the two groups were found. Again, we hypothesize that there was substantial overlap in the dependent variables of interest between the two groups.

MULTIGROUP COMPARISONS

In Table 8–15 we present a parallel description of multigroup comparisons involving at least three groups. Overall, 66% of the studies reported differences inferentially. No particular association was apparent between sample size range and reporting a statistically significant inferential difference, although the number of studies examined (total = 23) was small.

Summary and Discussion

Overall, our analysis shows a limited integration of statistics into the psychiatric nursing research literature. The articles examined showed a lack of sophisticated designs, absence of statistical references, small sample sizes, and infrequent use of inferential statistics.

Some characteristics of authors may be briefly cited, especially in relation to time trends. The majority of authors were nurses (69%) and the overwhelming majority of first authors were nurses (84%) as well. Although the percentage of doctorally prepared nurse authors remained constant from 1970 to 1985 (45%), the percentage of master's-prepared authors (42% overall) rose from 28% to 45%. With the increasing numbers of master's-prepared authors, it is not surprising that nearly one third (29%) of authors conducted the research in partial fulfillment of their academic degree requirements.

Most of the studies were conducted with minimal external support, as 83% lacked external (federal, state, local or private) funding. For most studies this probably limited the number of subjects that could be included in the study. It probably also limited the type of design and data-collecting methods that could be employed.

Although the mean number of references per study (article) was 17, the mean number of statistical references per study was only 0.2. Fewer than one article in five cited a statistical reference. This may imply greater familiarity of authors with the psychiatric nursing and the social science literature. This finding also suggests that the authors may not have been aware of valid options for study designs and analysis and/or may not have had access to statistical consultation.

About one third of the articles had a sample size range of 1–25; one third, a sample size range of 26–75; and one third, a sample size range of greater than 75. These generally small sample size ranges are consistent with the general lack of external funding and with the number of studies performed as part of the requirements for an academic degree.

Several other design characteristics are consistent with, and probably a consequence of, minimal external funding for the studies reviewed. Cross-sectional studies, which are generally less costly to perform than longitudinal studies, predominated in our analysis. Descriptive designs were more common than either quasi-experimental or experimental designs. Multivariate and multigroup study designs were only occasionally used.

Many of the investigators operated at an initial disadvantage because of lack of external funding or minimal resources. The consequence is small sample size and simplicity of designs. Many of the studies examined should have used inferential procedures but did not and could not because of small sample sizes. When investigators nonetheless attempted an inferential test, they were apt to obtain nonsignificant findings because of the small sample size.

In spite of the fact that the majority of studies had limited samples, a number of them did involve inferential statistical procedures and did report statistically significant differences in groups. Studies with standardized instrumentation were more apt to detect statistically significant differences, undoubtedly because of the more sensitive and reliable nature of the standardized instrument.

Detecting significant differences in groups was, surprisingly, not related to sample size. Instead, an examination of articles showed that population differences were large in those studies that detected differences and were minimal in those that did not. We need to recognize the obvious bias here that manuscripts reporting statistically significant results are more likely to be accepted for publication.

An important point is a comparison of the findings of this survey of the psychiatric nursing research literature with a study reported in the *New England Journal of Medicine*, which examined 71 clinical trials with negative findings in the medical literature (Freiman, Chalmers, Smith, & Keubler, 1978). All 71 studies reported no statistically significant difference in the percentages of successes between treatment and control groups, thus accounting for the fact that they were referred to as "negative trials." However, examination of the width of the confidence intervals for differences in treatment versus control percentages (most of which were based upon small sample sizes) revealed that it was uncertain whether the lack of significance resulted from lack of treatment efficacy or whether it resulted from small sample size. Thus, although the 71 papers reported no differences, the question of whether there were any differences could be argued either way. The important point here is that the psychiatric nursing research literature is within the same bounds of sophistication of previous research done using biostatistical procedures.

Recommendations

A major implication of this analysis is that the conduct of nursing research is difficult without funding. It makes for small sample sizes and for weakened power of the design and analysis. The thrust of the following recommendations is to increase sample size, as well as the sophistication of study designs and statistical analyses.

Whenever a study is contemplated, all sources of funding should be explored. Many of the investigators in this survey appeared to be new investigators, several having a master's degree as the highest degree earned. Nevertheless, local and small sources of "in-house" funding are frequently available and should be pursued. Another possibility is for new investigators to collaborate with more senior investigators, for example, by taking a small part of a larger project. An encouraging fact, and one that should promote psychiatric nursing research at the grassroots level, is the existence of specific funding programs for junior investigators at the federal level.

A second key issue in developing the psychiatric nursing research literature involves collaboration of investigators in multicenter and cooperative endeavors. Investigators in various sites could collect data according to a common protocol in examination of the same research question. Such a design would allow for larger sample sizes, which subsequently would allow for a more sophisticated design and quantitative analysis. It also would increase the generalizability of the findings.

Another form of collaboration is to have graduate students in nursing (master's and Ph.D.) collaborate in research to fulfill academic requirements for a thesis or dissertation. Far too often now the theses and dissertations are conceptualized in isolation from other investigations. In many cases the sample sizes of the isolated studies are minimal, leading to negative findings. A more productive approach would be to conceptualize several studies that are guided by a single research purpose and to collect data from different settings or different populations. Such an approach would again allow for larger samples, greater clarity of conceptual background, more subsets or groups, and a more sophisticated quantitative analysis.

A third key issue involves statistical consultation. Statistical consulting is a key concern to statisticians. Within the American Statistical Association and the Biometric Society, various sections encourage presentation of papers on practical issues of statistical consulting. One example is a book on statistical consulting by Boen and Zahn (1982), which discusses the need for a statistical consultant to develop a good "data-side" manner.

Our experience as consultants has shown us that the most common mistake of a consultee is showing up at the consultant's office and asking a question that should have been considered at an earlier time. The result is often that some decisions about design and quantitative methods have irretrievably damaged the integrity of the study and have lessened the ability of the study to answer the original research question. A commonly quoted humorous version of this dilemma involves the investigator who comes to the statistical consultant with a sample of four rats and is seeking statistical advice about how to divide the four mice into five groups.

In sum, the state of the integration of quantitative science into psychiatric nursing is both encouraging and discouraging. It is encouraging in that it is within the parameters of research integration in other fields involving applied statistics. It is less encouraging in an absolute sense in that the designs are often simplistic, sample sizes are small, and quantitative procedures are uncomplicated.

REFERENCES

Beyer, W. H. (1971). *Basic statistical tables*. Cleveland: Chemical Rubber Co.

Boen, J. R., & Zahn, D. A. (1982). *The human side of statistical consultation*. Belmont: Lifetime Learning Publications.

Devore, N. E. (1979). The relationship between previous elective abortions and postpartum depressive reactions. *Journal of Obstetrics and Gynecological Nursing, 9*, 237–240.

DiVasto, P. (1985). Measuring the aftermath of rape. *Journal of Psychosocial Nursing and Mental Health Sources, 23*(2), 33–35.

Fleiss, J. L. (1982). *Statistical methods for rates and proportions* (2nd ed.). New York: Wiley.

Fleiss, J. L., Tytun, A., & Ury, H. K. (1980). A simple approximation for calculating sample sizes for comparing independent proportions. *Biometrics, 36*, 343–346.

Freiman, J. A., Chalmers, T. C., Smith, J. Jr., & Keubler, R. R. (1978). The importance of beta, the type II error, and sample size in the design and interpretation of the randomized control trial: Survey of 71 'negative' trials. *New England Journal of Medicine, 299*, 690–694.

Gehan, E. A. (1980). The training of statisticians for cooperative clinical trials: A working statistician's viewpoint. *Biometrics, 36*, 699–706.

Gibson, D. E. (1980). Reminiscence, self-esteem, and self-other satisfaction in adult male alcoholics. *Journal of Psychiatric Nursing and Mental Health Services, 18*(3), 7–11.

Huck, S. W., Cormier, W. H., & Bounds, W. G. (1974). *Reading statistics and research.* New York: Harper & Row.

Keppel, G. (1973). *Design and analysis: A researcher's handbook.* Englewood Cliffs, NJ: Prentice-Hall.

Kerlinger, F. N. (1973). *Foundations of behavioral research.* New York: Holt.

Kirk, R. E. (1982). *Experimental design.* Belmont, CA: Brooks/Cole.

Lachan, R. (1982). Systematic sampling: A critical review. *International Statistical Review, 50*, 293–303.

Mosteller, F. (1981). Evaluation requirements for scientific proof. *Computing Biomedical Literature*, 103–122.

Murphy, S. A. (1984). After Mount St. Helens: Disaster stress research. *Journal of Psychosocial Nursing and Mental Health Services, 22*(9), 9–18.

O'Fallon, J. R., Dubey S. D., Salsburg, D. S., Edmonson, J. H., Soffer, A., & Colton, T. (1978). Should there be statistical guidelines for medical research papers? *Biometrics, 24*, 687–695.

O'Toole, A. W. (1981). When the practical becomes theoretical. *Journal of Psychosocial Nursing and Mental Health Services, 19*(12), 11–19.

Polit, D., & Hungler, B. (1983). *Nursing research: Principles and methods* (2nd ed.). Philadelphia: Lippincott.

Rosner, B. (1982). *Fundamentals of biostatistics.* Boston: PWS Publishers.

Shor, S., & Karten, K. (1966). Statistical evaluation of medical journal manuscripts. *Journal of the American Medical Association, 195*(13), 145–150.

Thibodeau, L. A. (1980). Evaluating selecting criteria. *Proceedings of the Statistical Association: Social Statistics*, 283–284.

Virgo, J. A. (1977). A statistical procedure for evaluating the importance of scientific papers. *Library Quarterly, 47*, 415–430.

Comment

The Search for Logic in Psychiatric–Mental Health Nursing

REG ARTHUR WILLIAMS, Ph.D., F.A.A.N.

As the story goes, a rather inebriated individual was searching under a lamp post for his house key that he had lost some distance away. A person observing this asked why he was not looking for the key where he had dropped it. He responded, "Because it is lighter here." Kaplan (1963), in *The conduct of inquiry: Methodology for behavioral science*, referred to this as the "principle of the Drunkard's Search" in searching for logic in the behavioral sciences.

Chapter 8 may suggest that psychiatric nursing from at least 1970 to the present may have been conducting research where the light was better, but not necessarily where the key may be found. The review of the psychiatric nursing literature revealed that the typical research article was published by a nurse in a psychiatric clinical journal with 1.9 authors. The journal author was likely to have a doctorate, but the study was not supported by external research funds. Further, a typical psychiatric nursing study had a clear statement of the problem but did not utilize a theoretical framework. The sample usually involved only one group with only 13 subjects, on average. The methodology most commonly employed was a cross-sectional design, but analysis was descriptive. Moreover, it involved only analysis of a single variable, and if inferential statistics were utilized, it usually was univariate. Finally, the typical article had 17 references. The need for increased sample sizes, more power to the design and analysis, as well as increased sources for external funding to accomplish these aims is well supported in the preceding chapter.

I would be remiss, however, if I agreed with all aspects of the points made. For example, the articles reviewed were limited to a traditional definition of psychiatric nursing, and those that addressed psychosocial aspects of nursing care were omitted. According to Fagin (1981), one of the strivings and achievements made by psychiatric nursing was the change of title to psychiatric–mental health nursing. This grew out of the combining of two distinctly different backgrounds in nursing, namely, psychiatry and public health. Although understandable, the narrow view of psychiatric nursing adopted in the preceding chapter may have excluded many studies that would have changed the overall characteristics of a typical research article in the psychiatric–mental health nursing domain. It would make an interesting study in itself to compare the results in Chapter 8 with a broader psychiatric–mental health nursing definition using journal articles examining psychosocial issues.

Only a third of the articles were found to have a theoretical framework, yet two thirds of the articles had clear statements of the problem. Since the problem is defined by the conceptual or theoretical framework, the authors–researchers of the articles must have had a clear notion of where things were heading. Fox (1982) defined a conceptual framework as "the ideas, understanding and research findings that provide both the foundation on which, and the background within which, research would be done" (p. 31), whereas a theoretical framework will utilize a theory to "organize and explain how some or all of the various relevant concepts are related" (p. 31). I would venture a guess that many of the articles reviewed did have a conceptual framework but not necessarily a theoretical framework. However, the authors give a number of good recommendations, such as increasing sample sizes, exploring all sources of funding; consulting with a statistician, and promoting nursing research through funding programs aimed at the junior investigator, just to name a few.

To address the problem of inadequate or inappropriate utilization of statistics, Gardner, Altman, Jones, and Machin (1983) have suggested statistical guidelines in preparing manuscripts for publication. Gardner et al. (1983) specifically developed a checklist to evaluate the statistical completeness of a paper as well as its acceptability for publication. An interesting point in this checklist is whether a statistician was involved as an author or acknowledged for help.

In examining statistics in psychiatric nursing, we must raise the question, "Are we being too hard on ourselves?" Our colleagues in medicine have identified similar concerns (e.g., Hartung, Cottrell, & Griffin, 1983; Longnecker, 1982; Mainland, 1984a, 1984b; Stanley & Pace, 1983). Boyer (1984), concerned about using just simple statistics in a medical journal, emphasized that "if we wish to advance the boundaries of knowledge, we must be able to ask and investigate questions in a way that does justice to the complexities of nature" (p. 659). Yet Emerson and Colditz (1983) found that 58% of the research articles appearing in the *New England Journal of Medicine* used no statistical methods or only descriptive statistics. By adding the use of the *t*-test, 67% of the articles were accessed, and by adding contingency tables, nearly three fourths of the articles were accessed.

Before a discipline can advance, it must describe in detail the phenomena it explores. Since psychiatric nursing has so many areas yet to describe, we might follow Kaplan's (1963) principle of the drunkard's search—examine our logic and research questions where the light is best, at least for now.

References

Altman, D. G., Gore, S. M., Gardner, M. J. & Pocock, S. J. (1983). Statistical guidelines for contributors to medical journals. *British Medical Journal, 286,* 1489–1493.

Boyer, W. F. (1984). Statistical analysis in The New England Journal of Medicine. *New England Journal of Medicine, 310,* 659.

Emerson, J. D., & Colditz, G. A. (1983). Use of statistical analysis in The New England Journal of Medicine. *New England Journal of Medicine, 309,* 709–713.

Fagin, C. M. (1981). Psychiatric nursing at the crossroads: Quo vadis? *Perspectives in Psychiatric Care, 19,* 99–106.

Fox, D. J. (1982). *Fundamentals of research in nursing.* Norwalk, CT: Appleton-Century-Crofts.

Gardner, M. J., Altman, D. G., Jones, D. R., & Machin, D. (1983). Is the statistical assessment of papers submitted to the "British Medical Journal" effective? *British Medical Journal, 286,* 1485–1488.

Hartung, J., Cottrell, J. E., & Giffin, J. P. (1983). Absence of evidence is not evidence of absence. *Anesthesiology, 58,* 298–300.

Kaplan, A. (1963). *The conduct of inquiry: Methodology for behavioral science*. New York: Harper & Row.

Longnecker, D. E. (1982). Support versus illumination: Trends in medical statistics. *Anesthesiology, 57*, 73–74.

Mainland, D. (1984a). Statistical ritual in clinical journals: Is there a cure?—I. *British Medical Journal, 288*, 841–843.

Mainland, D. (1984b). Statistical ritual in clinical journals: Is there a cure?—II. *British Medical Journal, 288*, 929–931.

Stanley, T. H., & Pace, N. L. (1983). Statistics should support rather than strangle anesthesiology literature. *Anesthesiology, 58*, 297–298.

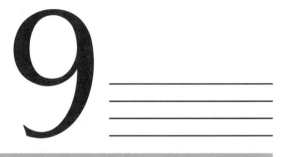

Statistics and Quantitative Methods in Community Health Nursing Research

BEVERLY C. FLYNN, Ph.D., R.N.

The Elaboration Model
Applications of the Model to Community Health Nursing
Research
Conclusions
Comment: Scientific Challenges in Community Health
Nursing

This chapter includes a generic framework for data analysis—the elaboration model (Lazarsfeld, Pasanella, & Rosenberg, 1972; Babbie, 1983)—and argues its applicability to research in community health nursing. The argument to support this model is based upon considerations of the state of the art in community health nursing (Highrighter, 1977, 1984) and the research approaches predominant in this domain of nursing (Flynn, 1984).

A major goal in nursing research is to increase the methodological and statistical adequacy of investigations. However, it is impossible to accomplish this goal without considering the content of the research in terms of the questions asked and the conceptual frameworks invoked. In this chapter, I hope to show that the use of the elaboration model enhances the scientific merit of research in community health nursing.

The Elaboration Model

The elaboration model is a logical framework for the analysis and interpretation of the relationships between two variables through the controlled introduction of other variables. The value of the elaboration model is that it aids in understanding the relationships between three or more variables, while being statistically simpler than more refined quantitative methods, like analysis of covariance and multiple regression modeling. The model allows the investigator to develop hypotheses and conduct further data analyses related to these hypotheses within the same body of data. Babbie (1983) notes that while ex post facto hypothesizing is invalid in science, researchers should be able to suggest reasons or a rationale for observations that do not confirm prior hypotheses. The elaboration model allows for this.

There are four basic steps in the elaboration model. The first is that a relationship between two variables is observed. Second, a third variable, called a "test variable," is held constant, in the sense that the cases under study are subdivided according to the attributes of that third variable. Next, the original two-variable relationship is recomputed within each of the subgroups to determine the partial relationships among the variables. Finally, the comparison of the original relationship with the partial relationship found within each subgroup allows a fuller understanding of the original relationship itself.

There are several guidelines to be considered in following these steps. To begin with, the analyst needs to know or hypothesize whether the test variable is antecedent or prior in time to the other two variables or whether it is intervening between them. This can be represented schematically as follows:

Antecedent Test Variable

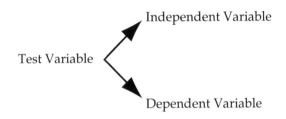

Independent Variable

Test Variable

Dependent Variable

Intervening Test Variable

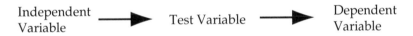

Independent Variable ⟶ Test Variable ⟶ Dependent Variable

The different positions suggest different logical relationships in the multivariate model. In the first case, the antecedent test variable affects the "independent" variable as well as the "dependent" variable. The terms *independent* and *dependent* are in quotations, because, as Babbie (1983) explains, the test variable is in fact the independent variable, and the other two are dependently related to the test variable. However, in this paper, we use the terms only to provide continuity with the examples in this chapter.

Since in the antecedent case the independent and dependent variables are both related to the test variable, a logical relationship to each other can be inferred. Yet it should be noted that this relationship is not causal. Instead, in the elaboration model it is assumed that the relationship between independent and dependent variables results from coincidental relationships to the test variable. The relationship is said to be spurious. If the test variable is intervening, the independent variable affects the test variable, which in turn affects the dependent variable.

Possible outcomes of analyses using the elaboration model are labeled *replication, explanation, interpretation,* and *specification* and provide different implications for understanding the original relationship. As the term suggests, *replication* means that the partial relationships are essentially the same as the original relationship, regardless of whether the test variable is antecedent or intervening. This replication of results gives support to the notion that the original relationship is a genuine one. *Explanation* describes a spurious relationship between the two original variables. The original relationship is explained away through the introduction of the test variable. Here the test variable must be antecedent to the other two variables and the partial relationships must be significantly less than originally found. *Interpretation* means that the intervening variable helps to interpret the mechanism through which the relationship occurs. It can be concluded that the original relationship was genuine and that the independent variable influences the intervening variable, which, in turn, influences the dependent variable. *Specification* means that the conditions under which the original relationship occurs are delineated regardless of whether the test variable is antecedent or intervening.

In essence, the elaboration model provides researchers with a step-by-step logical framework within which to specify empirical findings. Without such a framework researchers may fail to elucidate findings adequately that would prove or disprove the hypothesis, and thus be likely to make Type I and Type II errors.

Applications of the Model to Community Health Nursing Research

In this section the elaboration model is applied to selected studies in community health nursing to demonstrate its relevance to the field. I will highlight two studies that, perhaps by intuition, utilized the logic underlying the elaboration model. I will also present three studies that could expand the specificity of their research findings through further analysis of data using the elaboration model. It should be recognized that the researchers of these three studies may have conducted some of the analyses to be suggested but did not report the findings. If this is the case, I offer apologies to those involved, yet still contend that even the negative results of such findings are useful to report in order to provide further insights about the phenomena under study.

The first study that used the logic underlying the elaboration model is a classic community survey of health needs of the elderly to determine the implications for public health nursing services at the DuPage County Health Department in Illinois (Managan, Wood, Heinichen, Hoffman, Hess, & Gillings, 1974). This study did not test hypotheses, but it described the non-institutional elderly population by comparing the demographic characteristics of this population to their health needs in a step-by-step, logical manner. The major variables of interest are specified as follows:

Demographic Characteristics	Health Problems
Age	Health condition
Education	Physical functioning
Sex	Accessibility of medical care
Birthplace	Social isolation
	Service needs

First, each of the five parameters representing health problems was analyzed univariately. Next, bivariate analysis was conducted to compare these five health problems with the four demographic variables. Finally, one of the health problems, or a combined parameter of health problems, was used as a test variable in subsequent contingency analyses to indicate whether the demographic characteristics of the population having these health problems could be more specifically identified. For instance,

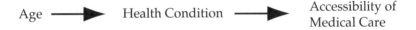

Age ⟶ Health Condition ⟶ Accessibility of Medical Care

In other words, one parameter of a health problem variable (health condition) was used as an intervening test variable between an independent demographic variable (age) and another dependent health problem variable (accessibility of medical care). Doing so permitted replication of the findings, interpretation of the mechanism through which the relationships occurred, and specification of the conditions under which the original relationship occurred.

The second study that used the logic of the elaboration model was a study of school nursing services for children with high absenteeism (Long, Whitman, Johansson, Williams, & Tuthill, 1975). This study hypothesized that children with frequent absences who received nursing services would have fewer absences from school. Bivariate analyses and matched pairs *t*-tests were used to compare the mean absences of children in the absenteeism group and the comparison group. Several demographic variables were used as intervening test variables between the independent and dependent variables:

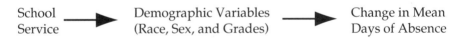

School Service ⟶ Demographic Variables (Race, Sex, and Grades) ⟶ Change in Mean Days of Absence

This study was another example of utilizing the thinking underlying the elaboration model for analysis and interpretation of relationships among the variables. The analyses clarified replication, explanation, interpretation, and specification identified in the elaboration model.

Three studies in community health nursing found in the literature are reviewed in terms of suggestions for further specificity in the findings. The first study examined the relationship between the complexity of patient care and the quality of care provided by community health nurses (Sienckiewicz, 1984). This study revealed no significant differences between control and experimental groups of patients. Although the author indicated that demographic data were collected on patients, these variables could have antecedent and intervening effects on the independent and dependent variables; for instance,

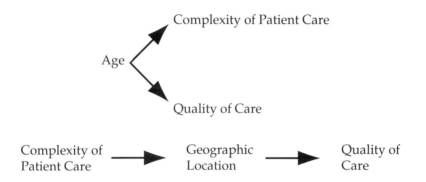

Babbie (1983) notes that when an original relationship is zero, the elaboration model can be used to identify the effects of a suppressor variable. The suppressor variable is one that conceals the relationship between the variables of interest. Thus, the elaboration model is applied to specify relationships that did exist but that were not evident in previous analyses.

The second study analyzed selected correlates of job performance of community health nurses (Koerner, 1981). The only significant association with job performance found was the state board examination score in surgery, and this was a negative association. The logic behind the elaboration model may explain this outcome of predominantly null results. The model of relationships among the variables described in the article could be revised to indicate alternative logical relationships. For example, perceived leadership style of nursing supervisors could be viewed as an intervening variable between state board examination scores in surgery and job performance:

State Board Examination   Leader   Job
Scores in Surgery   ⟶   Behavior   ⟶   Performance

Similarly, highest level of education could be viewed as an antecedent test variable to the state board examination scores in surgery and job performance:

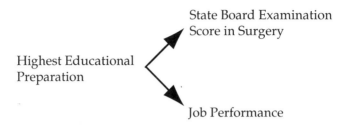

State Board Examination
Score in Surgery

Highest Educational
Preparation

Job Performance

The third study reported on the effectiveness of public health nurse postpartum home visits (Barkauskas, 1983). This study found no significant differences between home-visited and not-home-visited mother–infant pairs, except for the variable of concerns about health. It was concluded that "public health nurses can no longer afford to look upon the home visit as a general therapeutic event" (Barkauskas, 1983, p. 579). Multivariate contingency tables and two-way analyses of variance techniques were used to analyze the data.

A number of variables in the study could be introduced as test variables, either as antecedent to or intervening between the independent and dependent variables. For example, age of mother could be viewed as antecedent to the independent variable related to home visit and to the dependent variable concerns about health:

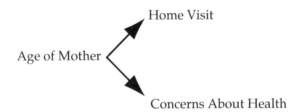

Home Visit

Age of Mother

Concerns About Health

Analyzing these relationships would indicate if the original relationship found could be replicated or whether it should be explained as a spurious relationship. It might also specify the conditions under which the original relationship occurred.

Another dependent variable of interest was postpartum health problems. If this variable was viewed as intervening between home visits and concerns about health, it could be assessed whether the findings could be replicated, further interpreted, and specified:

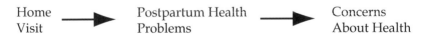

| Home Visit | Postpartum Health Problems | Concerns About Health |

These examples demonstrate the utility of the elaboration model to selected examples of research in community health nursing. They also demonstrate that data analysis should follow a logical pattern in order to maximize the understanding of the data, as well as the applicability of the elaboration model as a form of ex post facto data analysis. Theoretical formulations for nursing can be best accomplished through the elaboration model approach.

Conclusions

This chapter concludes with some priority areas of research in community health nursing. These areas are consistent with priorities for nursing research established by the Cabinet on Nursing Research of the American Nurses' Association (1985), the consensus conference on public health nursing practice and education (Lewis, 1985), the social policy statement of the American Nurses' Association (1980), and priorities indicated in World Health Organization documents on primary health care and nursing (International Council of Nurses & World Health Organization, 1979; World Health Organization, 1978, 1982, 1985).

It is obvious from the lay and professional literature that trends in American health care are changing community health care practice. Perhaps one of the obvious trends is the expansion of hospital-based services in the community and a proliferation of for-profit community health services (Starr, 1982). The result is that health care needs of particularly vulnerable groups in society—such as the elderly, the poor, persons from diverse cultures, and isolated persons—are left to the not-for-profit sector. These organizations are often without the resources needed to meet these needs in effective, accessible, and acceptable ways. A priority for community health nursing is the design and evaluation of alternative models for delivering community health care that incorporate both quality and cost effectiveness in meeting the nursing needs of these identified populations.

Because of the complexities of community health phenomena, there are many advantages to using qualitative along with quantitative methods in community health nursing research (Goodwin & Goodwin, 1984; Pelto & Pelto, 1978; Ruffing-Rahal, 1985). Using both methods in a single study can increase the meaning of data, help identify unanticipated consequences, and enhance the reliability and validity of the study.

The utilization of the elaboration model of data analysis for greater familiarity of the data's meaning is advocated prior to the use of more sophisticated multivariate statistical analyses. The elaboration model can also be applied in comparing data obtained from qualitative and quantitative methods of data collection.

In community health nursing research, there has been a proliferation of small, isolated studies that may have a number of untoward consequences for the profession. Ketefian (1975) noted these consequences as (1) a lack of cumulative knowledge as basis for practice, (2) a lack of programmatically oriented research, and (3) a lack of replication. It was rewarding to note that some efforts have been made to pull together information about isolated studies in an organized way in order to synthesize existing knowledge (Fagin, 1982; Highriter, 1977, 1984). Fagin's (1982) focus on the cost effectiveness of nursing through the compilation of 10 years of research on community care as an alternative to hospitalization is an excellent example of efforts that should be made in bringing together a body of knowledge on a priority area for research.

A final priority is that research needs to be focused on preventing or minimizing behaviorally and environmentally induced health problems that are major concerns to the community or society at large. Implied here is the involvement of community people themselves in the various phases of research, from identifying major community research needs to using results of research to improve community health. It is here that the results of research become part of the political process and thus can have a positive impact on health policy formation. Research findings need to be disseminated not only to community health nurses, but also to the general public and health policy makers. Although these groups may use the findings in different ways, all share the common denominator of being focused on policy making, whether in administrative, legislative, or judicial arenas. This way the utilization of nursing research can reach its maximum potential.

REFERENCES

American Nurses' Association (1980). *Nursing: A social policy statement*. Kansas City, MO: The Association.

Babbie, E. (1983). *The practice of social research*. Belmont, CA: Wadsworth.

Barbauskas, V. H. (1983). Effectiveness of public health nurse home visits to primiparous mothers and their infants. *American Journal of Public Health, 73*, 573–580.

Cabinet on Nursing Research, American Nurses' Association (1985). *Directions for nursing research: Toward the twenty-first century*. Kansas City, MO: The Association.

Fagin, C. M. (1982). The economic value of nursing research. *American Journal of Nursing, 82*, 1844–1849.

Flynn, B. C. (1984). Action research framework for primary health care. *Nursing Outlook, 32*, 316–318.

Goodwin, L. D., & Goodwin, W. L. (1984). Qualitative *vs.* quantitative research or qualitative *and* quantitative research? *Nursing Research, 33*, 378–380.

Highriter, M. E. (1977). The status of community health nursing research. *Nursing Research, 26*, 183–192.

Highriter, M. E. (1984). Public health nursing: Evaluation, education, and professional issues, 1977 to 1981. *Annual Review of Nursing Research, 2*, 165–189.

International Council of Nurses & World Health Organization (1979). *Report of the workshop on the role of nursing in primary health care*. Geneva: The Council and Organization.

Ketefian, S. (1975). Problems in the dissemination and utilization of scientific knowledge: How can the gap be bridged? In S. Ketefian (Ed.), *Translation of theory into nursing practice and education*. New York: New York University.

Koerner, B. L. (1981). Selected correlates of job performance of community health nurses. *Nursing Research, 30*, 43–38.

Lazarsfeld, P., Pasanella, A., & Rosenberg, M. (Eds.). (1972). *Continuities in the language of social research*. New York: Free Press.

Lewis, E. P. (Ed). (1985). *Collaboration in nursing education, practice, research*. Rockville, MD: U.S. Department of Health and Human Services.

Long, G. V., Whitman, C., Johansson, M. S., Williams, C. A., & Tuthill, R. W. (1975). Evaluation of a school health program directed to children with history of high absence. *American Journal of Public Health, 65*, 388–393.

Managan, D., Wood, J., Heinichen, C., Hoffman, M., Hess, G., & Gillings, D. (1974). Older adults: A community survey of health needs. *Nursing Research, 23*, 426–432.

Pelto, P. J., & Pelto, G. H. (1978). *Anthropological research: The structure of inquiry* (2nd ed.). Cambridge: Cambridge University Press.

Ruffing-Rahal, M. A. (1985). Quantitative methods in community analysis. *Public Health Nursing, 2*, 130–137.

Sienkiewicz, J. I. (1984). Patient classification in community health nursing. *Nursing Outlook, 32*, 319–321.

Starr, P. (1982). *The social transformation of American medicine*. New York: Basic Books.

World Health Organization (1978). *Primary health care: Report of the International Conference on Primary Health Care (Alma Ata, USSR, 6-12 September 1978)*. Geneva: The Organization.

World Health Organization (1982). *Nursing in support of the goal Health for All by the Year 2000*. Geneva: The Organization.

World Health Organization (1985). *A guide to curriculum review for basic nursing education*. Geneva: The Organization.

Comment

Scientific Challenges in Community Health Nursing

JEAN GOEPPINGER, Ph.D., R.N.

Researchers in the area of community health nursing face five challenges that are most pertinent to the advancement of the field. It is in this regard important to assess how statistics and quantitative methods can both facilitate and impede approaches and responses to these challenges. The five challenges are (1) the lack of definition of the domain of community health nursing; (2) the difficulties of operationalizing some key concepts; (3) the limited extent to which research in the community can be controlled; (4) the renaissance of interest in community care settings, such as the home and workplace; and (5) the application of research findings to practice and health policy shaping that practice. Obviously, not all of these challenges are unique to research in community health nursing. Just as noticeable is the observation that many of these challenges cannot be met with quantitative solutions alone.

The domain of community health nursing is unclear. We even define *community* differently, as (1) the setting of our practice and scholarship; (2) the unit of practice, the aggregate, or interacting group; and (3) the target of practice (Sills & Goeppinger, 1985).

I can personally attest to the difficulties of responding to the challenge of defining the domain. I spent three years (1979–1982) collaborating on an approach to the assessment of community competency (Goeppinger & Baglioni, 1985). We adopted a workable, if unused, definition of the rural community—that area bounded by telephone exchanges—and automatically lost all the potential respondents who did not have telephones or were not listed in the directory. So with one win and one loss we move ahead. We developed our initial assessment approach by painstaking and time-consuming Q-sorts using experts in community nursing, research, and practice. Then we moved on to some sophisticated computer applications, namely, cluster and factor analyses. We identified a simple four-factor model for examining the community as an interacting group and described a promising, practical approach to the assessment of community competence. The findings were not published until December of 1985 (Goeppinger & Baglioni, 1985). No nursing journal was interested in the substance of the research. Consequently, our contribution to clarification of the domain of community health nursing may be compromised.

Not all key concepts in community health nursing, should we ever agree on them, are readily amenable to measurement. Community health nursing research is a psychometrician's nightmare. In our investigation, the list of concepts that were difficult to operationalize was long. Already mentioned was *community*; add to this *community leader, natural helper, rural, function,* and *pain among persons with arthritis.*

It is in the operationalization of concepts that the computer and careful quantitative analyses can be helpful. We dealt with the measurement issues surrounding the concept of *community* by a series of factor analyses and are now working with similar methodologies on the concepts of *function* and *pain.* We are ignoring problems in the measurement of *natural helper* and *community leader* and we have decided to take an ethnographic approach to the definition of *rural.* We are convinced that some of our research must be carried out at the descriptive or factor-isolating level (Dickoff, James, & Wiedenbach, 1968). For example, neither the Census Bureau's nor the Department of Agriculture's definition of *rural* approximates the Virginians in our study, who live and work on the farms and in the farm-related industries of the Blue Ridge Mountains, the Shenandoah Valley, and the Piedmont Plateau.

The preceding chapter implicitly acknowledged the major challenge in community health nursing research with which statistics and quantitative methods can help: the need for control. Since field experiments are not all that common in community health nursing, control is achieved primarily through quasi-experimentation and the comprehensive collection and post hoc statistical analysis of data. The elaboration model in Chapter 9 is standard sociological practice and, in fact, is the basic logic of survey research. There are, however, limits to this type of analysis. The number of variables that can be handled is quite small, and the extent to which the effects of time can be ascertained is limited. Multiple regression models and time-series analysis, for example, permit more thorough and precise study.

Instrumentation can also add to the ability to "control" the richly complex research settings proper to community health nursing. Let me illustrate with an example from a current project on the impact of arthritis self-care education for rural persons. The original design was a pretest–posttest control group experiment. Rural persons with arthritis who volunteered to participate in community-based self-care education were to be randomly assigned to either a home-study–correspondence course, a small group, or a delayed treatment. Although the rigor of the design was undoubtedly a major factor in receiving several years of extramural funding, the apparent rigor of the design made me a bit nervous. As a community health nurse I know a bit about community life, especially community life in rural areas, having grown up in the country and worked largely in rural settings. People talk, and they do so in churches, at the grocery store, and at the farm sales resulting from bank foreclosures. Thus, the randomly assigned participants were bound to contaminate each other, and the design would be "blown." I sought consultation from a sociologist colleague at the University of Virginia (Biggar, 1983), who advised me: "You've been hanging around with psychologists too much! No self-respecting sociologist worries about contamination. Study the phenomenon but examine it as diffusion of information." A new research question was thus added to the project, namely, "Which method of self-care education is associated with the most extensive and in-depth diffusion of health information?"

There is a present renaissance of interest in community care settings accompanied by a commitment to use research findings to guide practice and shape research. Some of the inherent challenges are less readily solved via statistics and quantitative methods than others. Perhaps all that can be said is that we must continue to define the field of community health nursing, compete successfully for the research dollars (e.g., in the areas of prospective payment, ambulatory health care, and self-care), and then energetically disseminate scientific findings to fellow researchers, practitioners, and policymakers.

References

Biggar, J. (1983). Personal communication. Charlottesville: University of Virginia.

Dickhoff, J., James, P., & Wiedenbach, E. (1968). Theory in a practice discipline, Part 1. Practice oriented research. *Nursing Research, 17*, 197–203.

Goeppinger, J., & Baglioni, A. J. (1985). Community competence: A positive approach to needs assessment. *American Journal of Community Psychology, 13*, 507–523.

Sills, G. M., & Goeppinger, J. (1985). The community as a field of inquiry in nursing. *Annual Review of Nursing Research, 3*, 3–23.

10

Statistics and Quantitative Methods in Gerontological Nursing Research

ANN L. WHALL, Ph.D., F.A.A.N.
DOROTHY BOOTH, Ph.D., R.N.
MARY M. JIROVEC, Ph.D., R.N.

Gerontological nursing research is at least as old as the research in the other clinical areas of nursing if it is measured by the publication of gerontological nursing studies in nursing research journals. For instance, the first edition of *Nursing Research* included a gerontological nursing study. Just as other clinical areas in nursing have demonstrated increasing sophistication in research methodology and statistics, so has the field of gerontological nursing. However, this clinical specialty suffers from a major disadvantage. Until recently there were very few graduate programs in gerontological nursing. The fact that investigators in this clinical area have continued to conduct research, without widely based graduate education programs, is therefore something of a wonder. What is reported here is remarkable in and of itself, regardless of comparisons with other clinical areas.

Gerontological nursing research, for the purposes of this chapter, are those studies conducted by nurses that address the health and well-being of older adults. In this chapter we review statistics and quantitative methods in the research literature in gerontological nursing. We sampled a representative portion of the research in this domain of nursing so as to identify the quantitative statistical analyses used and to judge the appropriateness of these analyses. This review does not address research design and sampling, as other reviews have done (Brimmer, 1979; Brower & Crist, 1985; Gunter & Miller, 1977; Kayser-Jones, 1981; Robinson, 1976; Wolanin, 1983).

To examine the major compilations of, and hence a most representative sample of, this research, a decision was made to survey two journals: *Nursing Research* and the *Journal of Gerontological Nursing*. This decision was made because the former journal was the first nursing research journal and would thus demonstrate changes in the types of quantitative methods used in research over time. The latter was chosen because, since its first publication in 1975, it has been devoted to the publication of gerontological nursing research.

The term *quantitative methods* is operationally defined to mean quantitative statistical methods or the use of those statistical procedures that seek to quantify and measure, through some count method, some conceptual property or variable. The studies found in the two chosen journals that were indexed or otherwise identified as pertaining to aging or gerontology were examined for the types of statistical methods used. It is recognized that gerontological nursing studies are also found scattered throughout other, more recently published nursing journals, but to demonstrate a progression of statistical methods over time, the journals with longest standing in publishing gerontological nursing research (i.e., *Nursing Research* and *The Journal of Gerontological Nursing*) were chosen. It is also recognized that nurses publish in journals other than gerontological journals.

The method used in this survey was to identify studies as gerontological in nature through the journal indices or tables of contents and then to identify the major types of statistical methods used in these studies. Abstracts and briefs were not reviewed, because great variability was found in the reporting of statistical methods in these sources. Decisions needed to be made in the interpretation of the types of statistical methods used in studies for a variety of reasons. An *F* value, for example, was sometimes reported without alluding to the statistical procedure used to determine it. In other cases, fleeting reference might be made to, for example, a linear regression analysis, but the major discussion might center upon percentages. In these cases an effort was made to identify the major analyses that were used. Therefore, the results of this survey are considered representative of the statistical procedures used in gerontological nursing research; however, it should be noted that interpretations of the statistical procedures used were necessary.

An effort was made to categorize statistical procedures in a manner that might assist in understanding the level of sophistication exemplified by the use of quantitative methods. Consequently, descriptive versus inferential statistical procedures were identified, and inferential techniques were further divided into univariate versus multivariate statistical procedures. Descriptive statistics were defined for the purposes of this chapter as the use of percentages, and the use of measures of central tendency and dispersion to report the data. Although correlation, chi-square, and certain nonparametric procedures may at times be considered descriptive, these types of analyses were identified separately because of an increase in the complexity of these analyses over, for example, percentages. Univariate and multivariate analyses, for the purposes of this paper, are defined according to Harris (1975).

Chronological Overview

In reporting the findings of this survey, the results are reported in summary form, except in a few instances. Summaries are used so as to better demonstrate trends in the use of quantitative statistical methods in gerontological nursing research.

1950–1959

Only one gerontological nursing study was found in *Nursing Research* for the decade of 1950–1959. The article was found in the first edition of *Nursing Research* in 1952. In this study, Mack (1952) used both descriptive and inferential statistics. Multiple variables were considered but were not handled using multivariate statistics. Thus, a norm of relative sophistication was established at an early date by this study. Unfortunately, no other studies followed in the 1950s and many of the studies that followed were not as sophisticated in the use of quantitative procedures as Mack's (1952) study.

1960–1969

Five gerontological nursing studies were found in *Nursing Research* from 1960 to 1969. These studies included reports of the program of research by Schwartz (1960; Schwartz, Wang, Zeitz, & Goss, 1963). One study (Van Drimmelen & Rollins, 1969) on oral hygiene agents used more than descriptive and/or qualitative statistics (content analysis). These researchers used analysis of variance with post hoc analyses using Duncan's multiple range. Another study (Adams, Baron, & Caston, 1966) was not indexed under geriatrics but definitely met the criteria of gerontological nursing research. This study used chi-square analysis as well as descriptive statistics. Failure to classify this study as geriatric in the index of *Nursing Research* demonstrates an information retrieval problem.

1970–1979

Nineteen gerontological nursing studies were identified in *Nursing Research* from 1970–1979. Only three studies used primarily descriptive statistics to analyze the data. On the other hand, four used multivariate statistics (e.g., multiple regression analysis or MANOVA).The other studies used primarily *t*-test, correlation, or chi-square. The year 1979 found 10 gerontological nursing studies reported in *Nursing Research*, and none of these studies used primarily descriptive statistical procedures alone.

It was also in this decade that the *Journal of Gerontological Nursing* began to be published. Twenty-five studies were found between 1975 and 1979 in this journal, of which 19 used primarily descriptive analyses. The most frequently used descriptive technique was that of percentages. However, *t*-test, correlation, and ANOVA were also used, but much less frequently than percentages. There was one instance in which multiple regression analysis was applied.

1980–1985

Several gerontological nursing studies were found in *Nursing Research* between 1980 and June 1985. Of seven articles indexed as pertaining to aging for the years 1980–1984 two used multivariate statistical procedures. None used primarily descriptive statistics. The others used such procedures as correlation, ANOVA, and chi-square.

In the *Journal of Gerontological Nursing* between 1980 and June 1985, multiple gerontological nursing studies were found. Out of 64 studies reviewed, nine used multivariate statistics, mostly percentages, to report the data. The other studies used primarily correlation, analysis of variance, and chi-square.

Trends in the Use of Statistics and Quantitative Methods

Two important trends are evident from this review. The first trend is that the number of studies in gerontological nursing has increased over the decades. The second trend is the increasing sophistication that is evident in the use of quantitative statistical procedures. In *Nursing Research* in the 1960s, articles were published that used primarily percentages, means, and other descriptive procedures. In the 1970s this continued to be the case, although less so, with only three such studies being identified. In the present decade none of the studies in this journal used only descriptive analyses.

Publications in the *Journal of Gerontological Nursing* also reflect these trends. Whereas in the publications of the 1970s three fourths used primarily descriptive techniques, in the 1980s only one third used primarily descriptive statistics. In addition, the increased use of multivariate techniques is demonstrated in both journals. For the 1950s and 1960s, in *Nursing Research*, only one study with a multivariate technique was found. However, in the 1980s approximately one third of the articles in this journal used multivariate techniques. In the *Journal of Gerontological Nursing* the use of these techniques increased from about 4% in the 1970s to about 14% in the 1980s.

There is a danger, however, of concluding from this discussion that more complicated analyses are always best or appropriate at all stages of research development or for all types of studies. This conclusion is untenable, for in the early stages of inquiry descriptive studies are needed to identify the magnitude and scope of problems. Once the question of existence of a problem is answered affirmatively, studies may explore various aspects and approaches to the problem. At this stage inferential statistics are generally used. Once various aspects of the problem are identified through exploratory and/or descriptive studies, studies that control for and handle multiple variables are needed. At this point multivariate analyses are generally considered appropriate.

In gerontological nursing research this type of progression is evident. The widespread use of descriptive analyses from the 1950s through the 1970s is reflective of work toward the identification and exploration of various aspects of problems. The use of more advanced quantitative statistical procedures, such as those found in *Nursing Research* from the latter 1970s to the present time, is reflective of more advanced comprehension of the complexity of problems in gerontological nursing. The current use of path analysis techniques, for example, demonstrates a concern for theoretical model building, which is only possible after one has identified the nature and complexity of a variety of related variables. The use of ANCOVA as well demonstrates concern for multidimensional problems and situations.

The *Journal of Gerontological Nursing* demonstrates a slightly different pattern from that exhibited in *Nursing Research*. This journal continues to present studies that use primarily descriptive statistics. Because this journal publishes a large number of clinical studies, it is concluded, at least in part, that clinical research in gerontological nursing continues to be in a phase of development that in some proportion is descriptive–exploratory. This seems appropriate, given the magnitude of clinical problems in aging and the short history of nursing research in this area.

There is a concern, however, that the number of related and replication descriptive studies remains low. To stay at the descriptive level without attempting to interrelate this knowledge will adversely affect both clinical practice and theory development in the area of gerontological nursing and will foster a "bits-and-pieces" approach to the development of a clinical knowledge base. Descriptive research must now be interrelated and used as a basis for intervention studies and theoretical model building.

As graduate educational programs continue to prepare nurses in gerontological nursing research, the advancement of research in this area will continue. In particular, it is posited that there will be less use of univariate procedures, that instead investigators will move to multivariate techniques and procedures for handling multiple variables at one time. As clinical problems become better described and related interventions more often explored, multivariate analyses will be more appropriately employed and will in a very real sense be necessary.

Gerontological nursing research in the past has been reviewed and analyzed at least five times, and perhaps as many as eight times. This is an amazing amount of attention and self-analysis focused upon a relatively new (in an educational program sense) clinical area in nursing. Reviews have been conducted by Robinson (1976), Gunter and Miller (1977), Brimmer (1979), Kayser-Jones (1981), Wolanin (1983), and Brower and Crist (1985). Conclusions drawn in these reviews are relevant for the discussion here. It was discovered, for instance, that there is little replication of studies. This finding supports the need for not only the continued description of problems, but also examination of one study in relation to other studies. These reviewers also identified the need to draw inferences regarding specific population groups and the need to decrease purely descriptive work and use more advanced statistical procedures. In essence, these reviewers acknowledged the need for basic descriptive studies while at the same time suggesting that if gerontological nursing stays at this level, it will not contribute meaningfully to the field and the health care of older adults. Because persons are by nature complex and have been identified as the proper subject matter of nursing, and because the elderly most often have complex health needs, it would seem that suggestions from these reviews could be extended to the incorporation of multivariate statistical procedures. Although acceptance of this suggestion will not alter the nature of basically flawed research designs, it would assist in understanding the nature of the complex phenomena at hand.

Conclusion

This chapter took as its point of departure the need for graduate programs in gerontological nursing that prepare researchers in advanced research methodology to carry out the studies needed in this specialty area. Kayser-Jones (1981) commented that unless nursing does something about the quality and quantity of gerontological nursing education, the quality of nursing care for the elderly will suffer, at a time when the elderly are the fastest-growing segment of the population. This comment is relevant for the research produced in and by this specialty area. Unless nursing prepares graduate students in gerontological nursing to carry out research with sophisticated quantitative methods and statistical analyses, the acceptance of the suggestions presented here is in question.

References

Adams, M., Baron, M., & Caston, M. (1986). Urinary incontinence in the acute phase of cerebral vascular accident. *Nursing Research, 15,* 100–108.

Brimmer, P. (1979). Past, present, and future in gerontological nursing. *Journal of Gerontological Nursing, 5,* 27–34.

Brower, T., & Crist, M. (1985). Research priorities in gerontological nursing for long-term care. *Image, 17*(1), 22–27.

Gunter, L., & Miller, J. (1977). Toward a nursing gerontology. *Nursing Research, 26,* 208–221.

Harris, R. (1975). *A primer of multivariate statistics.* Orlando, FL: Academic Press.

Kayser-Jones, J. (1981). Gerontological nursing research revised. *Journal of Gerontological Nursing, 7,* 217–223.

Mack, M. (1952). The personal adjustment of chronically ill old people under home care. *Nursing Research, 1,* 9–30.

Robinson, L. (1976). Gerontological nursing research. In I. Burside (Ed.), *Nursing and the aged* (pp. 655–666). New York: McGraw-Hill.

Schwartz, D. (1960). Nursing needs of chronically ill ambulatory patients. *Nursing Research, 9,* 185–188.

Schwartz, D., Wang, M., Zeitz, L., & Goss, M. (1963). Problems of ambulation and traveling among elderly, chronically ill ambulatory patients. *Nursing Research, 12,* 165–171.

Van Drimmelen, J., & Rollins, H. (1969). Evaluation of commonly used oral hygiene agents. *Nursing Research, 18,* 327–333.

Wolanin, M. (1983). Clinical geriatric nursing research. *Annual Review of Nursing Research, 1,* 75–99.

Comment

Increasing Rigor and Meaningfulness in Gerontological Nursing Research

KATHLEEN COEN BUCKWALTER, Ph.D., R.N.

The field of gerontological nursing is characterized by steady growth and refinement, and this holds for practice as well as research. The preceding chapter underscores the strength of this evolution in its observations that an increasing number of gerontological nursing studies have been reported in *Nursing Research* and in the *Journal of Gerontological Nursing* and that the sophistication in quantitative statistical procedures applied to these studies has increased. It is striking, however, that the authors find the existence of gerontological nursing studies to be remarkable, given the paucity of graduate programs with a focus on aging, which limits the pool of nurses prepared to conduct gerontological nursing research.

It is true that more academic programs are needed and that the nursing profession must indeed improve both the quantity and quality of gerontology programs. However, other mechanisms currently exist that suggest we can expect the number of rigorous and meaningful gerontological nursing studies to increase, perhaps dramatically, in the near future.

First, nurse researchers with divergent clinical backgrounds are now becoming attracted to gerontological nursing and are conducting research on aging-related issues. Second, there are postgraduate and postdoctoral opportunities at the federal level to develop a research career in aging, and increasingly, nurses are taking advantage of these opportunities. For instance, the National Institute of Mental Health offers postdoctoral academic and faculty development awards in geriatric mental health, as does the National Institute on Aging. These awards encourage doctorally prepared nurses with research potential to redirect their clinical, educational, and research foci to gerontological issues. Second, the federal agencies that sponsor these awards offer assistance in proposal development and grant writing to nurse researchers. This increasing federal interest in and support for gerontological nursing research creates opportunities for nurses to obtain the extramural funding necessary to conduct larger and more sophisticated studies and thus to contribute to the noted trend of increased empirical sophistication.

Thus, although graduate education in gerontological nursing remains in need of development and expansion, we might predict a growth in research that is faster than the growth of graduate education. This research will come from a growing cadre of doctorally prepared nurses with a variety of clinical backgrounds.

It is also most likely that this research will not be published solely in the nursing literature. For as the authors of the preceding chapter well recognize, gerontological nurse researchers do not limit their publications to the two journals surveyed in this chapter. Some of the most significant gerontological research currently under way is conducted by nurse principal investigators, who head multidisciplinary research teams and who publish their findings in journals with a broader aging focus (e.g., *Gerontologist, Journal of Gerontology*) or in journals where their results may better impact on a particular target audience (e.g., *Journal of the American Geriatrics Society*). In general, these journals mandate more rigorous methodological approaches and sophisticated analytical techniques for acceptance of a manuscript than is required by the *Journal of Gerontological Nursing*. Moreover, these journals offer a forum for theoretical model building, replication studies, and practice concepts, which the authors note is so essential to gerontological theory development and practice.

Increased application of more advanced statistical techniques to gerontological nursing studies, the second trend noted in the preceding chapter, is certainly appropriate, given the complex and multidimensional focus of much of this research. The use of multivariate statistical instead of descriptive techniques is certainly needed to advance our understanding of gerontological phenomena as applied to theory and practice. However, this needs to be considered in light of selected characteristics of the elderly population under study. Indeed, the frail, dependent, and vulnerable nature of many of our elderly subjects can prohibit the effective and justified use of certain statistical techniques. For example, in our research related to increasing communication ability of elderly institutionalized aphasics, attrition by death, transfer to an acute facility, or onset of another disabling illness accounted for an almost 40% loss of the original sample over a three-year period. This censored data set precluded some of the more advanced analyses initially planned. Similarly, many studies on aging use self-report response formats that may not be usable with cognitively or sensorily impaired older adults, the severely debilitated, or aphasics.

Further, over the course of the study period, the fact that many of the elderly subjects were ill or dying greatly influenced their scores on the dependent measures, especially those related to patient satisfaction. Therefore, careful examination of individual raw scores and measures of central tendency and dispersion proved critical to understanding and interpreting the (skewed) data. We then created dummy variables to account for the health status of "outlier" elderly subjects (because of illness or imminent death) in order to get a more accurate picture of subjects' satisfaction.

The perspective that few of the clinical problems and research questions encountered in the elderly are unidimensional needs to be emphasized as much as possible. Similarly, it is important to highlight again that statistical analyses that manage multiple outcome and predictor variables are appropriate for many gerontological studies and are essential to advance our understanding of gerontological issues and the development of a data-based practice with older adults. We must also realize that quantitative methods may not always be best or even appropriate to investigate some of the phenomena of interest to gerontological nurses. The viability of other methodologies for selected gerontological nursing research topics should be recognized.

In conclusion, the scope of gerontological nursing research

must continue to broaden itself, as must the cadre of investigators in this field. The great diversity among the elderly compels investigators to develop a broad range of methodologies and statistical approaches to gerontological nursing research questions. Yet, because of characteristics of the study population as well as those of the field of gerontological nursing, it is essential to recognize the potential relevance of qualitative approaches as well. It is perhaps the alternating or combined use of qualitative and quantitative methods that will allow investigators to preserve both richness and rigor in their data.

11

Research in Nursing Administration: A Nursing Diagnosis Approach to the Measurement of Nursing Care

EDWARD J. HALLORAN, Ph.D., F.A.A.N.
MARYLOU L. KILEY, Ph.D., R.N.

The ultimate goal of measurement in nursing is the ability to explain and predict the effect of nursing action. The establishment of a correspondence between the rules of measurement and observed nursing care is needed to accomplish this goal. In this chapter, we make a case for using nursing diagnosis as both a framework and measurement approach for administrative nursing research. We begin by exploring the nursing process as a referent of nursing care. This is followed by a critique of current methods for studying nursing work. Next we examine the validity and feasibility of measuring nursing process by means of nursing diagnosis. Finally, by linking nursing diagnosis with nursing demand and resource allocation measures, we demonstrate the feasibility of studying administrative issues in nursing within a context of cost (money).

Nursing Process

Yura and Walsh (1973) define the nursing process as an orderly, systematic manner of determining the client's problems, making plans to solve them, initiating the plan or assigning others to implement it, and evaluating the extent to which the plan was effective in resolving the problems identified. The nursing process was developed in response to an effort to depict nursing as more science than art. Steps in the nursing process parallel those used to describe the scientific method: assessment, planning, implementation, and evaluation. A cyclic, ongoing process is maintained where each step can occur with and influence the others.

While the importance of the nursing process to clinical care is generally accepted, it is less known that professional entities have adopted the nursing process perspective to govern their activities. The American Nurses' Association Standards for Nursing Practice (ANA, 1973) are based on the nursing process concept. The Joint Commission for the Accreditation of Hospitals (JCAH, 1984) emphasizes in its requirements for the organization of nursing services that the delivery of nursing care must rest on the concept of nursing process. Given both this clinical and structural interest in the nursing process, it is imperative that research in the organization and delivery of nursing services be focused on the nursing process.

The Measurement of Nursing Work

Measuring nursing work is a complex task, and a focus on the nursing process may make it even more complex. In a sense, nursing work defies quantification. Nurses individualize and humanize the nursing care they give to their patients. The nursing process stresses the uniqueness of individuals and their health needs. Given this personalized system of nursing care, it seems unlikely that givers or receivers of care can know in advance what care is indicated in a given situation. Yet two predictive methods for estimating nursing work (i.e., what needs to be done for an individual patient) have wide usage in nursing practice. It is important to assess the extent to which they truly measure nursing work from a perspective that is acceptable to nurses and nursing.

The first method is based on medical classification and incorporates a medical model. It predicts nursing care to be delivered to patients on the basis of their medical diagnosis or disease state or in reaction to a care regimen ordered by a physician. The second system is based on observations of what nurses physically do to and for their patients. This model emphasizes a conventional operations research perspective.

Neither of these methods incorporates a coherent and substantiated perspective on nursing. In the first model, nursing is conceived of as primarily dependent on a pathological process. It assumes that the observable work of nurses, especially in acute care settings, is a direct result of orders from a physician and that nursing is perhaps nothing else but following the proverbial "doctor's orders." In the second model, nursing care is described as a listing of nursing tasks, reflecting an underlying thinking that nursing care is an aggregate of operationally definable executions of tasks. It also implies that a list of all discrete tasks performed by nurses can be developed, which is most doubtful. Both types of systems further share a common disadvantage in that they were developed solely for classification purposes, and not for scientific measurement; that is, they were created to measure aspects of nursing work, and certainly were not designed to measure function of generalization, abstraction, and knowledge development.

The critique on the predominant focus on tasks and task execution does not imply that nursing care is not concerned with the physical components of patient care or that it occurs without interaction with the care provided by physicians (referred to as the dependent functions of nursing). However, there is an increasing emphasis on independent nursing actions, which encompass all facets of care from the physical aspects to counseling and teaching. The validity of any measurement approach to nursing work depends on the extent to which this perspective on independent and dependent nursing actions is fully acknowledged and integrated.

The existing approaches to the measurement of nursing work are strongly influenced by the conceptualizations and methodologies from disciplines other than nursing (e.g., economics, industrial engineering, management science). It seems that this has led to confusion between the means of the research and the desired ends. Although some of the quantitative thinking in nursing administration is, for example, from the basic economic theory of limited resources and unlimited demand, studies of economics related to nursing frequently are more concerned with testing an economic model than with realizing a solution to a nursing problem. This illustrates the difficulty of merging conceptualizations and methodologies from different disciplines so as to serve the purposes of one of these disciplines. It is therefore important that research on the nursing process be about the nursing process, not about a methodology to which the nursing process can be applied. The ideal, of course, would be to have conceptualizatons and methodologies that are specific to the discipline.

The development of such conceptualizations and methodologies should, moreover, take place within a conceptualization of nursing that is focused on the practice of nursing, and therefore amenable to observation in practice. There is meager evidence on the successful implementation of theoretical nursing models in practice settings. King (1971), Orem (1971), Rogers (1970), and Roy (1974), to name a few, have formulated nursing theories, but their use has been limited mostly to education and research. It is perhaps because these theories do not agree on an operational definition of nursing that successful implementations in practice have eluded them.

The Measurement of Nursing Process Through Nursing Diagnosis

We argue that nursing diagnosis can provide the framework for measuring the nursing process, whether it is for the purpose of organizing and delivering nursing services or for the purpose of generating knowledge and advancing nursing science. Of primary importance, then, is whether nursing diagnosis is a valid framework and whether nursing diagnoses are valid operationalizations of components of the nursing process.

The issue of validity is composed of the issues of relevance and reliability. The relevance of the proposed use of nursing diagnosis as a

REFERENCE TEST

CNS ASSESSMENTS

		Agree	Disagree	Total
RN ASSESSMENTS	Agree	434 Both agree diagnosis present	277 CNS says No RN says Yes	711
	Disagree	174 CNS says Yes RN says No	3999 Both agree diagnosis not present	4173
		608 Total Positive*	4276 Total Negative*	4884

*Assumes clinical nurse specialist is correct as the reference test.

Figure 11–1. Agreement on nursing diagnosis between registered nurse specialists in 4884 diagnostic opportunities.

framework and as a method is a matter of intellectual and scientific debate. This debate has been going on in both written and spoken forms, and closure and conclusiveness are not anticipated in the near future.

Our work in the past decade or so has yielded comparative data and reliability estimates that have contributed to our current view on the relevance of a nursing diagnosis approach. Through a first set of studies, we have shown that nursing diagnosis explains more of the variation in length of hospital stay than the DRG representation of medical diagnosis (Halloran & Kiley, 1985; Halloran, Kiley, & Nadzam, 1986; Halloran, Kiley, & Nosek, 1985).

A second set of studies focused on measuring the need for nursing care in order to model more accurately hospital utilization in the health care system (Halloran, 1980; Halloran & Kiley, 1983). Table 11-1 presents an example of nursing need described with nursing diagnoses in two independent samples. Although the samples in these studies were not examined for case mix and are convenience samples, they do demonstrate nursing need in a hospital and attest to the reliability of measurement. Indeed, the mean days of occurrence of 8 of 16 nursing diagnoses were within 99% confidence intervals. These eight diagnoses were disturbance in body image, sleep disturbance, excess nutrition, excess fluid volume, thought process alteration, urinary incontinence, bowel incontinence, and impaction.

Third, in a pilot study, Halloran (1976) explored the reliability of diagnostic ability of nurses (Topf, 1986). The applicability of 37 nursing diagnoses to patients during 66 patient days was evaluated by nurses. This provided 4884 diagnostic opportunities. The data are summarized in Figure 11–1. Sensitivity and specificity estimates were derived from these data. Sensitivity, the proportion of true positives correctly identified, was .71. The

TABLE 11–1. INCIDENCE OF NURSING DIAGNOSES WITH MEAN FREQUENCY OF OCCURRENCE DURING LENGTH OF STAY IN TWO INDEPENDENT SAMPLES*

Nursing Diagnosis	1980 Sample (n = 2560)		99% Confidence Interval	1983 Sample (n = 1294)	
	% of Cases	Mean Days Occurrence		% of Cases	Mean Days Occurrence
1. Discomfort	83.5	2.72	(2.60, 2.84)	79.9	2.50
2. Pain	45.9	1.83	(1.68, 1.98)	60.4	2.51
3. Nutrition depletion	35.2	1.81	(1.62, 2.00)	40.3	2.29
4. Disturbance in body image†	28.9	1.80	(1.61, 1.99)	35.4	1.93
5. Sleep disturbance†	28.2	1.68	(1.49, 1.87)	20.0	1.52
6. Bowel elimination: constipation	26.3	1.51	(1.39, 1.63)	31.4	1.86
7. Decreased cardiac output	23.9	2.66	(2.42, 2.90)	9.4	1.48
8. Excess nutrition†	19.1	1.78	(1.55, 2.01)	11.3	1.81
9. Fluid volume deficit	16.7	1.55	(1.31, 1.79)	31.8	1.81
10. Excess fluid volume†	13.2	1.89	(1.58, 2.20)	24.1	2.10
11. Bowel elimination: diarrhea	13.2	1.65	(1.38, 1.92)	21.6	2.10
12. Thought process alteration†	8.6	2.29	(1.86, 2.72)	12.6	2.03
13. Urinary elimination: retention	8.3	1.49	(1.15, 1.83)	21.9	1.88
14. Urinary elimination: incontinence†	4.6	1.90	(1.38, 2.42)	13.8	2.28
15. Bowel elimination: incontinence†	3.4	2.32	(1.68, 2.96)	9.7	2.53
16. Bowel elimination: impaction†	1.3	1.37	(0.59, 2.15)	3.9	1.32

*Geometric means are used because of the skewed distributions of the variables due to length of stay (each observation was transformed to the logarithm to the base 10, the mean obtained, and the antilog obtained).

†Nursing diagnoses with mean days of occurrence within 99 percent confidence limits in two independent samples.

specificity of nursing diagnoses, the proportion of true negatives correctly identified, was .93.

Nursing Process and Money: Measurement of Nursing Action for Resource Allocation

Delivering nursing services costs money. Surprisingly, however, administrative research in nursing has only recently begun to consider the variables of time and money, when in the reality of everyday management of nursing resources, costs have long been measured in terms of time and money. Both time and monetary scales fit the real number system and ratio level measurement. The importance of using money (and indirectly, time) as a common denominator is further underscored by the fact that this scale is the foundation of current economic and accounting systems and that it permits choices to be made among available alternatives for goods and services of equal monetary value. Rather than circumvent or criticize this system, it is essential that nurses actively participate in the choice of attributes to be measured that reflect a valid concept of nursing.

In Figures 11–2 and 11–3, two conceptualizations of the behavior of staffing and acuity relationships are presented, but each has different variables. In Figure 11–2 acuity is defined as the number of time and task units done, but in Figure 11–3 it is defined as nursing dependency units treated. Nursing dependency units are measures of nursing need derived from the average number of nursing diagnoses per patient day. Let us examine both conceptualizations as to their adequacy to describe the behavior of staffing acuity relationships, and, relatedly, the underlying concept of nursing.

In Figure 11–2, the use of time and task as the measures of nursing assumes that nursing care can be quantitatively represented as an additive linear function. Yet to what extent can nursing care really be broken down into time and task units? Does this not reflect a view of nursing criticized earlier as dominating the classification systems? It can be argued indeed that nursing care consists of simultaneous, multiple actions (and effects of these actions)—for instance, reassurance, hygiene, and surveillance all at the same time. Because of the simultaneity of multiple items, a multiplicative, nonlinear function is indicated to describe the relationship between nursing demand and the staffing required to meet that demand. An example of this function is given in Figure 11–3.

It is important to point out that, according to the model specified in Figure 11–3, we will not only be able to represent nursing demand more accurately (i.e., as nursing dependency units), but also be able to meet the existing demand with less staff. Assume that the function f(nurses) is to attain

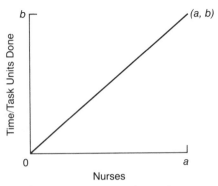

Figure 11–2. Linear relationship.

a desired coordinate (x,b) with x being the unknown. In Figure 11–2 this coordinate is attained by the value a. In contrast, in Figure 11–3, this coordinate is attained by the value a', which is smaller than a. Consequently, the value b, being the number of nurses to meet the nursing dependency, is attained with fewer nurses. The area between the function of time and task (dotted line in Figure 11–3) and the curve is the potential productivity of the nursing care delivery model over and above the time and task parameters. Note that this productivity is not absolute and therefore not a function of the number of nurses (i.e., expense) under all circumstances. A minimum number of nurses is always required on a ward, regardless of patient need, as long as one patient is hospitalized on that ward.

It should be clear that a time and task perspective fails in its measurement of nursing resources. Instead, as the models in Figures 11–2 and 11–3 show, nursing resources should be described in a form that incorporates what patients need, and how these needs may interact at any point in time.

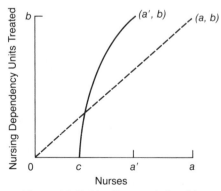

Figure 11–3. Nonlinear relationship.

Given the accumulating evidence on the reliability of nursing diagnoses as descriptors of patients and their needs, the growing support for the nursing diagnosis framework, and the fact that cost factors can be derived from nursing diagnoses, the endorsement of nursing diagnosis as a measurement approach to future administrative nursing research appears justified. With the current efforts also to explicate and taxonomize nursing interventions and nursing outcomes, the future of nursing administration research may indeed prove to be one of relevance and rigor.

References

American Nurses Association (ANA) (1973). *Standards of nursing practice.* Kansas City: The Association.

Halloran, E. J. (1976, October). *A process oriented nurse staffing methodology.* Paper presented at the 2nd Annual Nursing Research Conference of the Westside Veterans Adminstration Medical Center, Chicago.

Halloran, E. J. (1980). Analysis of variation in nursing workload by patient medical and nursing condition (Doctoral dissertation, University of Illinois at the Medical Center). *Dissertation Abstracts International, 41-09B.*

Halloran, E. J., & Kiley, M. (1983). The relationship between length of stay and nursing diagnosis. Unpublished raw data, University Hospitals of Cleveland.

Halloran, E. J., & Kiley, M. (1985). *Nursing dependence as an alternative measure to severity of illness measures complementing the DRG.* Unpublished manuscript, University Hospitals of Cleveland.

Halloran, E. J., Kiley, M., & Nadzam, D. M. (1986). Nursing diagnosis for identification of severity of condition and resource use. In *Proceedings of the Sixth Conference on the Classification of Nursing Diagnoses.* St. Louis: Mosby.

Halloran, E. J., Kiley, M., & Nosek, L. (1985). *Nursing complexity, the DRG, and length of stay.* Unpublished manuscript, University Hospital of Cleveland.

Joint Commission on Accreditation of Hospitals (JCAH) (1984). *Accreditation manual for hospitals.* Chicago: The Commission.

King, I. (1971). *Toward a theory for nursing.* New York: Wiley.

Orem, D. (1971). *Nursing: Concepts of practice.* New York: McGraw-Hill.

Rogers, M. (1970). *An introducton to the theoretical basis of nursing.* Philadelphia: Davis.

Roy, Sister Callista (1974). The Roy adaptation model. In J. P. Riehl & Sr. C. Roy (Eds.), *Conceptual models for nursing practice.* Norwalk, CT: Appleton-Century-Crofts.

Topf, M. (1986). Three estimates of interrater reliability for nominal data. *Nursing Research, 35*(4): 253–255.

Yura, H., & Walsh, M. (1973). *The nursing process.* Norwalk, CT: Appleton-Century-Crofts.

Comment

On Describing the Need, Process, and Outcome of Nursing Care

JERRY L. WESTON, Sc.D., R.N.

The following comments focus on three major themes that can be extracted from the preceding chapter. First, although the concept of nursing cannot be measured, the components of the nursing process can. However, and this is the second theme, whether the measurements have validity is open to question. And third from an administrative perspective, nursing diagnoses translate into the utilization of nursing resources that translate into money.

With regard to the first theme, the authors correctly point out that patient assessment forms the basis for the nursing process. Data collected are of two types: those reported by the patient and observations by the nurse of the physical needs and functional abilities of the patient (Adams, 1984; Hanchett, 1977). These data are then organized in a meaningful way for nursing actions. The first step in this organization is the nursing diagnosis.

Hanchett (1977) has indicated that, beginning in 1953, the literature referred to nursing diagnosis as the entire nursing process, including identifying nursing problems. According to this author, it was not until 1977 that the term *nursing process* came into use, with nursing diagnosis as one of the components. One could say that the vague terminology has never been fully resolved, and this may pose a problem in achieving Halloran and Kiley's laudable goal of measurement by nursing diagnosis. Indeed, nursing diagnoses appear to be the same as patients' presenting problems amenable to nursing interventions, as is demonstrated by the following definition by Gordon (1976): "Nursing diagnoses, or clinical diagnoses made by professional nurses, describe actual or potential health problems which nurses, by virtue of their education and experience, are capable and licensed to treat" (p. 1299).

There are other factors to be considered before fully adopting a nursing diagnosis approach to the measurement of nursing care. First, nursing diagnoses have a relatively short history compared with medical diagnoses, and there is something to be said for confirmation and consolidation over time. Not all nursing diagnostic categories are empirically validated, and those that are have not gone much beyond initial phases. Gordon (1982) remarked that although it is advantageous to have nursing diagnoses represent the diversity in nursing, "the disadvantage is that diagnoses are at various levels of abstraction and disparate in conceptual focus" (p. 312).

The examples of nursing diagnoses found in the preceding chapter reflect this lack of standardization. Although they are very similar to the North American Nursing Diagnosis Association (NANDA) classification, they have been adapted to the authors' institution. For instance, Discomfort and Pain are separate diagnoses, but NANDA uses a single diagnosis, namely, Comfort, Alterations in: Pain. This brings us to the issue that terms used to describe nursing care should clearly and specifically communicate the distinguishing features of nursing: the need for, the process of, and the outcomes of nursing care. The proposed labels for nursing diagnoses (e.g., impaired mobility and alterations in nutrition) attempt to identify the basis for nursing interventions (e.g., bed, bath, and feeding) and a fundamental necessity for an adequate description of nursing care.

The second theme, whether measurements of nursing process have validity, is in need of further research. It can be argued that in many cases the diagnosis is not a 0–1 dichotomy, but rather an interval or ratio type of scale that, if a problem is present, measures its intensity from 0. An example is the previously mentioned diagnoses of Pain and Discomfort. The point at which discomfort becomes pain is subjective; what is excruciating pain to one person may be severe but tolerable pain to another. The nursing demands of these people are most likely to differ. Also, discomfort and pain assessments may differ if the observer is a patient or a nurse.

The third and final theme consists of the double question of whether, from an administrative perspective, nursing diagnoses can be translated into (1) the utilization of nursing resources and ultimately (2) the measurement nearest an administrator's heart, money. The answer to the first half of the question might be negative, at least for most diagnoses. The diagnosis of Incontinence might lend itself to inferences about resource utilization. Yet as long as a dichotomous scaling method prevails, a diagnosis such as Impairment of Skin Integrity, where the degree is paramount, would not.

The authors' case for measuring nursing demand and nursing resource allocation on the basis of nursing dependency units is innovative. Yet it should not be forgotten that nursing acuity classifications based on the need of the patients' medical condition are receiving a great deal of attention with the expansion of prospective payment reimbursement or pricing systems. It will be important for nursing administrators and researchers in nursing administration to merge the interests of nursing with those of the health care system at large. It may be then that the understanding of the patterns of service intensity within and across case types will be understood and that innovative ways of establishing a foundation for organizing and delivering patient care will be assured.

REFERENCES

Adams, C. E. (1984). Nursing diagnosis in patient care planning. *Military Medicine, 149*, 202–204.

Gordon, M. (1976). Nursing diagnosis and the diagnostic process. *American Journal of Nursing, 76*, 1298–1300.

Gordon, M. (1982). *Nursing diagnosis: Process and application*. New York: McGraw-Hill.

Hanchett, E. S. (1977, September). *The problem-oriented system: A literature review*. U.S. Department of Health, Education, and Welfare Publication No. (HRA) 78-6, Health Resources Administration.

PART 3

Issues in the Integration of Nursing and Quantitative Science

12

Crossing Disciplinary Boundaries: Statistics, Quantitative Methods, and Multidisciplinary Inquiry

KAREN E. DENNIS, Ph.D., R.N.

Whether nurses cross disciplinary boundaries or conduct research independently, the strongest scientific studies evolve when investigators are expert in a specific substantive area of inquiry as well as in research design, instrumentation, and statistical analysis. When the roles of clinical researcher, quantitative scientist, statistician, and computer scientist are combined within one individual, the potential for a single study's contribution to scientific knowledge is unparalleled. However, the exponential increase in the number of studies conducted within the health care disciplines over the last 20 years, combined with advances in research design, statistics, and computer applications, virtually precludes one individual from having all the necessary knowledge for implementing the complex studies required to understand multidimensional phenomena.

It is an interesting yet troubling paradox that nurses are having to argue for the credibility and viability of nursing research while trying to integrate it into the mainstream of multidisciplinary inquiry. The uniqueness of nursing is emphasized when we demonstrate the critical role that nursing research has in building a knowledge base for nursing practice and in defining the contributions that nursing alone makes to the health of individuals. Nurse scientists can contend with the research design and analysis issues of multidisciplinary orientation by examining different models of collaborative research with other scientists.

Multidisciplinary Models

Multidisciplinary research commonly is considered to be the integration of knowledge and resources of individuals from more than one discipline in order to study problems that otherwise could not be addressed as effectively (Disbrow, 1983). Within that broad definition, however, there are as many multidisciplinary research models as there are investigators to implement them. Williams (1983) suggested that collaborative research and group research form the ends of a continuum characterizing projects with more than one investigator. She defined collaborative research as a democratic, cooperative endeavor among peers, while describing group research as several investigators working together on the same project. Interdisciplinary research projects can fit anywhere along the continuum from collaborative to group research and may shift positions repeatedly as they evolve.

In a scientific investigation involving more than one person, it is important to consider both structure and process. Although a treatise on the group dynamics of interdisciplinary research extends beyond the scope of this chapter, the willingness of several investigators to sit in the same room and work through ideas and issues is the foundational imperative. There are few publications on interdisciplinary group process as it pertains to research, but several nurses involved in such projects have shared their insights on some of the important issues (Bergstrom, Hansen, Grant, Hansen, Kubo, Padilla, & Wong, 1984; Disbrow, 1983; Krueger, Nelson, & Wolanin, 1978; Williams, 1983). The three following collaborative or group research models focus on structure more than process, reflect actual as well as potential multidisciplinary formats, and are illustrative rather than exhaustive of the possibilities.

NURSING: AN INTEGRATION OF MANY DISCIPLINES

Nurses with doctorates in physiology bring expertise in the measurement and analysis of physiological variables, and enrich the discipline with the use of multiple indicators in order to triangulate the phenomenon under investigation. Their research designs that translate cellular and organ functions into activities of daily living and clinical applications reflect and support nursing's holistic perspective.

Nurses with doctorates in psychology bring expertise in experimental designs that are important for assessing behaviors and the effectiveness of interventions. Issues related to random assignments to groups, internal and external validity threats, as well as univariate and multivariate analysis of variance in all their forms become familiar considerations in psychology-oriented nursing research.

Nurses with doctorates in sociology bring expertise in large-scale surveys and share with their colleagues the design, sampling, instrumentation, and analysis issues inherent in that methodology. Multivariate approaches, such as canonical correlation, factor analysis, discriminant analysis, and log linear analysis, can be used in these studies with large sample sizes without violating some of the assumptions of statistical tests and subject–variable ratios.

It is well recognized that physiology, psychology, and sociology are not the only disciplines to which nurses have turned for advanced educational preparation. When nurses with doctorates in all the related sciences and in nursing pool their knowledge and experience, there is a richness in diversity and a potential for multidisciplinary collaboration within nursing that is perhaps not found in other areas of inquiry.

INTEGRATING OTHER DISCIPLINES WITH NURSING

The number of studies with multiple authors published in four nursing research journals during the period 1977–1981 attests to the collaborative or group efforts undertaken by some nurse researchers. In 1977 and 1981 the number of single- and multiple-authored works was fairly equal, although ratios fluctuated in the intervening years (Moustafa, 1985). Although it usually is not possible to discern the disciplines of nonnurse investigators listed as co-authors, they presumably are experts in conceptual, measurement, and/or statistical components of the study or series of studies on a specified topic. In this model, the roles of clinician, methodologist, and statistician are divested in different individuals but find cohesion in the topic and the research questions.

When using this model for crossing interdisciplinary boundaries, nurse researchers share an approach common to investigators in all fields. The contributions of other scientists are elicited to strengthen research in one's own discipline rather than to blend interests and broaden the scope of a study or series of studies. However, "horizontal building" research, the investigation of complementary pieces of a theoretical area (Bergstrom et al., 1984), holds promise for increasing the visibility and viability to nursing research in multidisciplinary inquiry.

INTEGRATING NURSING WITH OTHER DISCIPLINES

To make a horizontal building model viable, a nurse researcher must be able to define and communicate the goals of nursing research, convince others of its importance, and juxtapose the interests of nursing research with those of other disciplines. Medicine is not the only discipline with which nursing engages in horizontal building research, for collaboration with nutritionists, exercise physiologists, and psychologists, among others, is also important. Nevertheless, it is necessary and obvious to consider a nursing–medicine interdisciplinary focus.

Despite the vast amount of research conducted within the field of medicine and the large amounts of money being channeled to it, only eight of the articles with multiple authors published during 1983–1984 in *Nursing Research, Research in Nursing and Health*, and *Western Journal of Nursing Research* included physicians as the nonnurse investigators. Reasons for the small number of nurse–physician research projects are many and are more tacitly understood than explicitly discussed. Both physicians and nurses acknowledge that the classic role of nursing in relation to physician research is implementing the medical protocol. Nurses interested in research either recognize that role and consciously choose it or adopt it as a matter of course in physician-dominated medical institutions. Perhaps nurse researchers have preferred not to attempt studies with physicians because they acknowledge the traditional perils or recognize impenetrable barriers. But the scientific community loses when these two critical health care disciplines fail to merge their efforts and expertise.

Nurses' collaboration with physicians is possible in any institution where physicians are conducting research, but general clinical research centers (GCRCs) offer an environment particularly conducive to multidisciplinary inquiry. Expanding its geographic ability to provide research facilities beyond the Clinical Center in Bethesda, Maryland, the National Institutes of Health, through its Division of Research Resources, funds GCRCs in major medical centers across the United States. The most recent directory (Division of Research Resources, 1984) lists 75 of these centers and their major areas of investigation. To date no centers have supported nursing research. Nursing research, as a GCRC major area of investigation, can be conducted independent of work by those in other disciplines as well as in concert with them.

Nurse researchers' participation in multidisciplinary inquiry involving physicians may take many forms. In the most familiar type, investigators may develop a protocol that measures variables of interest to both disciplines. Studies dealing with adherence–compliance, patient–provider relationships, or incontinence are a few limited examples conducive to this type of collaboration.

In another approach, nurses and physicians may become investigators on one another's protocols; some nursing research may coincide with a protocol being conducted by a physician to examine variables of concern to nursing that otherwise would remain unexplored. For example, a nurse researcher interested in extending and refining extant work on preparation for stressful medical procedures could form a link with a physician admitting patients for a study involving cardiac catheterization. The same subjects would be involved in both studies, but different variables would be examined; nurses and physicians would collaborate to implement both protocols.

In yet another structure, nursing research may span the protocols of several physicians, again looking at variables of concern to nursing. Nurses interested in examining certain preventive health behaviors across the life span may draw subjects from a variety of physicians' protocols and investigate such diverse phenomena as age-related changes in metabolic, endocrine, pulmonary, and cardiac function.

To any of these multidisciplinary forms, nurse researchers bring the strength of their broad-based methodological repertoires. Their knowledge of the design alternatives for investigating various problems, as well as issues pertaining to measurement and statistics that may be unfamiliar to investigators in other disciplines, enhances collaborative inquiry. On the other hand, perpetuation of the design, measurement, and analysis problems inherent in many nursing studies is also possible. Inadequate control over internal and external validity threats (Cook & Campbell, 1979), inattention to the reliability and validity of measures (Lynn, 1985; Waltz & Strickland, 1982), and inappropriate use of multiple t-tests to identify differences among treatment groups (Muller, Otto, & Benignus, 1983) cross interdisciplinary boundaries along with their conceptual counterparts.

Methodological Dilemmas

Collaborative inquiry has many strengths, but it also is replete with methodological dilemmas, which are magnified from the combined perspective of many disciplines. Researchers engaged in multidisciplinary, horizontal, scientific inquiry must ascertain that the theoretical areas being studied are complementary rather than conflicting and that study designs can deal with potentially diverse research questions and a proliferation of dependent variables. Difficult multidisciplinary issues arise throughout the development and implementation of a research project, but the elements of design, sampling, attrition, and analysis are particularly important to consider.

DESIGN

It is important to acknowledge that some disciplines believe "good science" can only be accomplished within the context of certain designs. Since many disciplines consider experimental designs to be *the* approach for ascertaining causal relationships, certain investigators may not accept alternative approaches, such as those involving causal modeling and path analysis. Indeed, they may not accept descriptive and exploratory designs at all, insisting instead that hypotheses be tested. Even within experimentation, some disciplines use small numbers of subjects who serve as their own controls in cross-over designs, whereas others use distinct treatment groups with pre- and posttesting (Disbrow, 1983). Developing several small studies within one major project, using different but compatible designs to answer the various research questions, and making pragmatic compromises are some of the possible solutions.

SAMPLING AND ASSIGNMENT

One study's heterogeneity may be another study's homogeneity, as differences in selection criteria are identified. One recognized way to eliminate the influence of an intervening variable is to exclude it from the study sample. Since there are certain gender-related differences in aging, for example, some investigators may want to exclude women from an experimental design examining the influence of an intervention on metabolic function. Other investigators who want to examine whether those interventions also influence a sense of well-being may seek to include persons from both genders. In the process of identifying participation criteria, these researchers must evaluate the impact of gender on both studies to reach a satisfactory decision. Regardless of the specific decision made, the sample size in this type of collaborative investigation must be large enough to provide an adequate subject–variable ratio and sufficient statistical power for both areas of inquiry.

Although clinical studies usually tend not to select subjects randomly from the total population of interest, those involving experimental designs do make random assignments to treatment groups. Although coin flipping and tables of random numbers are usual approaches to random assignment, a more efficient method for effecting randomization in large multidisciplinary studies is use of the random number generator found on most computer systems.

Assignment may become complicated, however, in the stratified randomization of subjects across protocols that interact. For example, an examination of the effects of different interventions targeted at decreasing subjects' anxiety may influence a variable being measured for another protocol featuring different age groups. Therefore, even though age may not be a pertinent stratification variable in one protocol, subjects may need to be stratified by age before being randomly assigned to interventions. In so doing, investigators can meet the scientific aims of both protocols without sacrificing the integrity of either one.

A word of caution is warranted at this point. Investigators must be careful that horizontal building studies support, rather than undermine, the objectives of each. Decisions must be made about whether to overlap studies and variables, or to proceed independently. Although the time, energy, and costs to be saved and the scope of knowledge to be contributed in overlapping protocols are tempting, it is not scientifically sound for any discipline to use whatever clinical population happens to be readily accessible. Inappropriate heterogeneity or homogeneity among subjects may jeopardize the internal and/or external validity of the studies involved.

ATTRITION

Attrition is a familiar and perennial problem of clinical trials where subjects are followed over a prolonged period of time. Although some nurse researchers may not have to contend with this issue because of the descriptive or cross-sectional designs of their studies, the loss of subjects from treatment groups in experimental research can lead to biased results.

As nurses build upon descriptive knowledge, move toward examining interventions that produce desired outcomes, and collaborate with other disciplines where experimental designs are more prominent, methodological and statistical ways of dealing with attrition will become increasingly important.

Five major categories encompass the reasons for attrition from clinical trials: (1) ineligibility discovered after enrollment; (2) noncompliance with the protocol related to changes in condition, side effects, loss of subject interest, or a variety of other reasons; (3) losses to follow-up due to death, subjects' transfer to another area, or failure to return for repeated measures; (4) competing events that pose as intervening variables undermining the determination of causal relationships; and (5) outliers (Friedman, Furberg, & DeMets, 1984). Some solutions to these problems are procedural. Mechanisms can be developed to ensure that all diagnostic data are received before enrollment decisions are made, to cross-check for transcription errors, and to maintain subjects' interest.

Other methods of dealing with attrition are statistical. Analyzing available data both with and without losses is one approach. If both analyses present similar findings, the interpretation is fairly clear. If results differ, then the interpretation must be made with caution. Reporting the results with all data included is perhaps the most valid, since that report most accurately reflects what was done in that particular study (Friedman, Furberg, & DeMets, 1984). Nevertheless, results may be conservative because of loss of power from the presence of ineligible subjects who would not have benefited from the treatment under any circumstances. Another statistical approach to the issue of loss is to undertake one of several forms of survival analysis.

Survival, or lifetable, analysis is used when subjects are entered into the clinical trial at different times and have various lengths of follow-up because of the termination of the study or other sources of loss (Friedman, Furberg, & DeMets, 1984). The Kaplan–Meier estimate (Kaplan & Meier, 1958), which uses conditional probabilities to estimate a survival curve across the entire study, necessitates knowledge of the exact time of entry into and loss from the clinical trial. With the Cutler–Ederer estimate (Cutler & Ederer, 1958), it is assumed that losses are uniformly distributed over a particular interval. A discussion of the specific calculations extends beyond the scope of this chapter, but it is important to note that computer programs are available to calculate survival data quite rapidly even for very large data sets.

DATA ANALYSIS

Issues related to procedures for the statistical analysis of data, already mathematically complex, are further compounded by the different types of data collected during the course of multidisciplinary investigations. In a study involving patients with diabetes, for example, physicians may examine the impact of exercise on glucose and fat metabolism; exercise physiologists may identify differences in aerobic versus nonaerobic exercise outcomes; nutritionists may explore the effects of trace elements and dietary fibers; and nurses may investigate factors influencing maintenance of self-care practices, including dietary control and leisure activity. The types of data collected, therefore, may include biochemical analyses on serum and cells, vital signs, measures of cardiovascular function, self-reported affective responses, and observational measures. Although the use of multiple measurements or triangulation is a strength of this study, the analysis of these types of data requires markedly different statistical procedures.

Nonparametric as well as parametric techniques, such as descriptive statistics, chi-square, paired comparisons, multiple regression, and analysis of variance, may be employed to answer the respective research questions. While investigators may be well versed in the statistical procedures required to analyze the types of data collected within their own disciplines, they may not be adept at thinking about analyses across interdisciplinary boundaries. For example, the physiologist who thinks in terms of means and standard deviations, frequencies, and paired comparisons may not be experienced with the use of factor analysis or the analysis of covariance common in psychosocial research.

For all investigators, the risk of inflating error rates in studies involving multiple variables looms large. Where the use of a t-test may have sufficed before, analysis of variance (ANOVA) may need to be used to control experiment-wise error rates. Investigators need to guard against the temptation to do multiple t-tests to compare group means, whether implemented in lieu of analysis of variance or after a significant F ratio is derived (Muller, Otto, & Benignus, 1983).

Indeed, even the use of analysis of variance in clinical trials has its limitations. Where multiple dependent variables are involved, multiple ANOVAs face the same error inflation as multiple t-tests. The multivariate analysis of variance (MANOVA) was developed to control the experiment-wise error rate of a large collection of univariate ANOVAs (Muller, Otto, & Benignus, 1983). MANOVAs, however, are seldom reported in the literature, perhaps because of the small sample sizes often used in clinical research and the distorted error rates that stem from violated assumptions. With multidisciplinary studies and the possibility of increased numbers of subjects, these complex multivariate procedures become more tenable.

Organizing Interdisciplinary Data

Analysis of voluminous data sets would have been next to impossible prior to the advent of the digital computer. With increasing numbers of statistical programs available for use on computers and with researchers becoming more knowledgeable about computers, data from these multidisciplinary studies can be input, stored, processed, and retrieved with relative ease.

McCormick (1983) identified four major categories of statistical packages, which reflect their intended use and capabilities: large, general-purpose statistical packages; statistical packages with more restricted applications; subroutines for special statistics; and database management packages. We refer to McCormick (1983) for a discussion of the first three categories and focus here on the fourth.

Of particular importance to researchers engaged in multidisciplinary work is the ability to organize and store diverse types of data upon collection and to retrieve them efficiently for different types of analysis. Database management systems are software programs that manage everything that happens to data from file definition and input, through analysis, to output (McCormick, 1985). Written in user-friendly English, database systems are available that use interactive queries and responses rather than researcher-generated procedural statements. These systems, therefore, are conducive to use by nonprogrammers and researchers who are not computer fluent.

An advantage of database systems is the format of data organization. Whether they are relational systems, which use common elements to link together two or more related structures, or hierarchical, with branches like an organizational chart, data can be displayed in conceptual frames. All data for an individual subject, data on one variable for all subjects, or data at one measurement period can be displayed. The researcher does not need an inordinately complex code book to isolate the variables of interest from a vast array of numbers. Although large statistical packages have "select if" statements that accomplish similar goals, database systems can handle a large number of specifications in a very efficient manner.

A disadvantage of the database system is its inability to perform some of the more complex statistical procedures appropriate for data collected on psychosocial variables. Although they can do some arithmetic functions and statistical analyses, these database procedures tend to be limited to descriptive statistics, chi-square, and univariate analysis of variance. For multivariate techniques, selected data must often be transferred and loaded onto a mainframe computer.

Conclusion

The advent of sophisticated statistical procedures and the development of complex computer programs to perform them have meant enormous progress in scientific inquiry. It is well known, however, that no amount of extensive statistical analysis and intricate computer programming can salvage a poorly designed and executed study. In addition, no hardware, software, or statistical formula can deal with the extraordinary complexities and sensitivities involved in group dynamics. As more nurse researchers become involved in multidisciplinary projects, different structures are needed to integrate their work on a myriad of topics, but the process has only just begun. Continued progress in this area will be brought about by the creativity and commitment of those scientists who choose to grapple with the personal, statistical, and methodological issues inherent in crossing disciplinary boundaries.

References

Bergstrom, N., Hansen, B. C., Grant, M., Hansen, R., Kubo, W., Padilla, G., & Wong, H. L. (1984). Collaborative nursing research: Anatomy of a successful consortium. *Nursing Research, 33*, 20–25.

Cook, T. D., & Campbell, D. T. (1979). *Quasi-experimentation: Design and analysis issues for field settings*. Boston: Houghton Mifflin.

Cutler, S., & Ederer, F. (1958). Maximum utilization of the lifetable method in analyzing survival. *Journal of Chronic Disease, 8*, 699-712.

Disbrow, M. A. (1983). Conducting interdisciplinary research: Gratifications and frustrations. In N. L. Chaska (Ed.), *The nursing profession: A time to speak*. New York: McGraw-Hill.

Division of Research Resources (1984). *General clinical research centers*. Bethesda, MD: National Institutes of Health.

Friedman, L. M., Furberg, C. D., & DeMets, D. L. (1984). *Fundamentals of clinical trials*. Boston: John Wright, PSG.

Kaplan, E., & Meier, P. (1958). Nonparametric estimation from incomplete observations. *Journal of the American Statistical Association, 53*, 457–481.

Kirk, R. E. (1968). *Experimental design*. Belmont, CA: Brooks/Cole.

Krueger, J. C., Nelson, A. H., & Wolanin, M. O. (1978). *Nursing research: Development, collaboration, and utilization*. Germantown, MD: Aspen.

Lynn, M. R. (1985). Reliability estimates: Use and disuse. *Nursing Research, 34*, 254–256.

McCormick, K. A. (1983). Data capture: Use of statistical packages and computer literature searches. In O. Fokkens (Ed.), *Medinfo-83*. Amsterdam: North-Holland.

McCormick, K. A. (1985). Computers in nursing research: Clinical, laboratory, statistical. In K. Hannah (Ed.), *Use of computers and information science*. Amsterdam: North-Holland.

Moustafa, N. G. (1985). Nursing research from 1977 to 1981. *Western Journal of Nursing Research, 7*, 349–356.

Muller, K. E., Otto, D. A., & Benignus, V. A. (1983). Design and analysis issues and strategies in psychophysiological research. *Psychophysiology, 20*, 212–218.

Waltz, C. F., & Strickland, O. L. (1982). Measurement of nursing outcomes: State of the art as we enter the eighties. In W. E. Field (Ed.), *Proceedings of the First Annual SCCEN Research Conference*. Atlanta: Southern Council on Collegiate Education for Nursing.

Williams, C. A. (1983). Establishing and implementing collaborative investigations. In O. L. Strickland & S. P. Damrosch (Eds.), *Proceedings of the Third Annual SCCEN Research Conference*. Atlanta: Southern Council on Collegiate Education for Nursing.

Comment

Theory Development Within an Interdisciplinary Context

CLAUDIA J. COULTON, Ph.D.

The preceding chapter has cogently pointed out the advantages and value of interdisciplinary research as well as some of the barriers to its implementation. It also touched on numerous issues in design and data analysis that are common to interdisciplinary research as well as to monodisciplinary research. Rather than add to this very comprehensive treatment, I would like to use experiences in interdisciplinary research to illustrate some of the issues identified.

Although I have been involved with numerous interdisciplinary projects over the past several years, there is one in particular that serves as a useful example. The project is focused on critical care and has brought together a diverse team, including persons whose primary interest is nursing care, health services research, health care financing, decision analysis, medical ethics, moral philosophy, statistics, and social sciences. One thing that has been clear in this mix is that interests, rather than discipline, have dominated role definitions. For example, I am a social worker and I asked social science questions. The psychiatrist had an in-depth knowledge of ethics and moral philosophy. Another nurse was interested in decision analysis. The administrator's interest had crossed numerous areas, as had the biostatistician's. Thus, one key to doing exciting and creative interdisciplinary research is to avoid rigid expectations. Discipline, profession, or position should not dictate who does what in terms of research activities. Overlapping of interest areas should be encouraged. Leadership on particular research questions or aspects of the study has been defined by interest and past experience, not by title. The conclusion to be drawn is that excessive efforts to define the role of nursing research, medical research, social work research, and others may actually be dysfunctional.

A second unique and beneficial aspect of this interdisciplinary project has been the varying perspectives and levels of analyses reflected in the research questions. Some of the analyses have focused on cost and public policy questions. Others have focused on clinical decision making. Yet the analyses related to public policy have been made richer through interaction with clinicians and administrators. The studies of clinical decisions have been assessed in terms of implications for public policy.

This experience of interdisciplinary collaboration also revealed what may be a limitation, or at least a major difficulty, in this type of research activity. This is related to the establishment of coherent theoretical frameworks to guide the study. Theories are made up of concepts and explanations of the relationships among those concepts. Theories are developed and tested by numerous scientists conducting investigations over a period of years and are typically associated with a single discipline. The same phenomenon can be conceptualized in several ways and embedded in several theories. When persons from various disciplines attempt to investigate the same phenomenon using alternative conceptualizations and theories, the risk is theoretical chaos and inappropriate mixing of units and levels of analysis. An example of this has arisen in our work regarding the question of whether a life-sustaining treatment is or is not implemented in critical care. If this is viewed using a theoretical perspective of psychological decision making, the focus would be on the decision makers' cognitive processes. Questions would be asked regarding judgments or probabilities and utilities. If the phenomenon were viewed from a sociological perspective, theories relating to social worth, social stratification, and group dynamics may be invoked. From an ethical perspective, moral theory related to autonomy, beneficence, and distributive justice may be primary. The concepts that would require operationalization and measurement differ widely in these approaches. The unit of analysis also differs—the psychological theory calls for a focus on the decision maker. The sociological theory focuses on the social relationship between the patient and decision maker. The ethical theory focuses on the patterns or relationships among decisions.

To achieve coherence in this situation, either one perspective is given primacy, theory is abandoned, or three studies are done. Too often theory is ignored, resulting in fewer theoretical contributions emerging from interdisciplinary research. A more desirable outcome would be deliberately and thoughtfully to combine or link theories, where possible.

13

Statistics, Quantitative Methods, and Grantsmanship: Methodological Adequacy of Research Grant Applications

MARY S. HARPER, Ph.D., F.A.A.N.

This chapter is focused on the development of research and the generation of knowledge through funded investigation. As in other disciplines, this is of importance to the full maturation of nursing research as a scientific discipline and its integration into the scientific community at large. This chapter presents advice on how to maximize the scientific merit of research grant applications. This is done by identifying problems generally encountered with research proposals and providing suggestions that have been found to enhance the quality of these proposals. Although the emphasis is on the federal funding system, much of this chapter can be extended to other sources of funding as well. Note that much of the content of this chapter is presented in the form of lists. The decision was made to emphasize practical application and, consequently, to present information in a format that promotes the development of proposals with a high probability of funding.

By means of introduction, it continues to be striking that, notwithstanding the tremendous increase in doctorally prepared nurses, the growth in nursing research activity has not been greater. Further, as an "observer" of the research movement in nursing and in my affiliation with one of the major federal funding agencies, it is of concern that little significant increase in the scientific merit of nursing research proposals is noticeable yet. Is this lack of emphasis in the quality of proposals due to a lack of quantitative methodology and statistics in some of the doctoral programs? Or is it because of the increase in nurses with doctorates in other disciplines who, in addition to being unable to meet the research standards of these disciplines, are not grounded enough in them to transpose related knowledge successfully to nursing? Whatever the reason, it is not uncommon to see proposals from nurses that are methodologically flawed, in addition to often being "half-baked-nursing" and "half-baked-other-discipline." Funding agencies are committed to nursing research, albeit perhaps to varying degrees; they will fund research that is nursing *and* meets general standards of scientific merit.

Distinguishing Funded from Unfunded Research Projects

Although the most obvious differences between funded and unfunded research projects are the scope and the availability of money, there are also a number of distinctions to be drawn related to proposal development and project execution. The following is a listing of distinctions, as well as implicit guidelines:

1. A proposal is written in response to the guidelines of the granting agencies, and these guidelines should be strictly adhered to. It is not uncommon for granting agencies to exclude from consideration any information and materials not in accordance with their guidelines.
2. Although multiple avenues for funding a particular research project exist, and many agencies might be interested, it is necessary to spend considerable time and effort in finding the appropriate funding source. This issue is addressed in greater detail later.
3. It is crucial to establish a relationship with the funding resource to determine better whether its priorities and interest are compatible with the ideas and aims of the proposal. Visiting agency staff for working meetings and sending project outlines to them are most helpful.
4. While the funding is there to be spent, often on a variety of activities and items, there are rules and policies that govern the allocation, spending, and transfer of budget items. Budgeting expertise is essential and consultation should be sought as necessary.
5. The federal funding agencies, but also many nonfederal ones, have specific human rights policies regarding the use of human subjects, freedom of information, and informed consent. Similarly, there may be policies involving civil rights—for instance, policies regarding affirmative action.
6. Awards are made to the institution or organization *in the name of* the principal investigator (or program director). Both the institution/organization and the principal investigator share responsibility for implementation of the project in keeping with designated policies, legislation, and mission of the funding agency.

Locating Sources of Funding

There are literally thousands of funding sources for research. These include federal, state, and local government agencies; private foundations;

business and industry; universities; private donors; and professional and scientific organizations. The federal government supports both extramural (nonfederal employee investigators) and intramural research (by federal employees at federal sites). Extramural research awards are made to both nonprofit and profit institutions and organizations, including corporations. In some of the health areas, certain foundations and private businesses are funding more research than the federal government (Kehrer, Aiken, Blendon, & Rogers, 1984).

A distinction is made between grants and contracts. Grants are awards to an institution or organization in the name of the principal investigator to assist the awardee in the conduct of research as specified in the proposal. Grants are initiated by principal investigators under the aegis of their institution or organization. Contracts, on the other hand, refer to the procurement of a product or service for use of the federal government. Typically, a research topic and the methods for conducting the research are specified in detail by the federal agency, although sometimes only general research guidelines are provided. In addition to contracts awarded after solicitation, some agencies also award contracts to unsolicited proposals. The availability of research contracts funds is announced through requests for proposals (the so-called RFPs), notices of which are published in the *Commerce Business Daily* and the *Federal Register*.

LINKING PROJECTS WITH POTENTIAL FUNDING SOURCES

From the beginning, it is important to explore the congruency between the financial resources of a particular funding agency and the budget demands for a project. Five major questions should be considered in locating a funding source:

1. Does the proposed problem or topic fall within the range of interests and priorities of the funding source, and can a cogent argument to that extent be made?
2. Does the funding agency provide the range of funds needed for project implementation?
3. Will the funding source be able to allocate money for the duration of the time needed to carry out the project?
4. Will the funding source consider co-funding the project with another public or private institution? This pertains to the funding of new projects and to whether the agency has regulations on parallel funding of related projects.
5. What are the limitations on the funding (e.g., funding of construction, renovation, and animal studies)?

STRATEGIES FOR LOCATING FUNDING SOURCES

Information on the availability of research funding can be obtained from five sources, and investigators should consult these in detail.

The *Catalogue of Federal Domestic Assistance* provides detailed descriptions of more than 100 federal programs. It contains three useful indexes. The Functional Index lists the government programs by interest areas (e.g., mental health, and education). The Subject Index contains the types of assistance by categories of services or selected beneficiaries. The Agency Program Index records the services that each federal government agency administers. The Catalogue describes each funding program in terms of the type of assistance offered, eligibility requirements, appropriations made, regulations, contact individual, and the names and addresses of regional and local federal offices that can be contacted for more information or application documents. This publication is available from the Superintendent of Documents, Government Printing Office, Washington, DC 20402, or from Federal Office Buildings in some cities.

The *Federal Register* is an invaluable daily publication that is modified throughout the year so that it provides the most up-to-date information about funds available from different federal programs. Also included in the *Federal Register* are new guidelines for programs, deadlines for grant programs, proposed changes in legislation and regulations, and composition of advisory committees. The *Federal Register* is available from the Superintendent of Documents, Government Printing Office, Washington, DC 20402.

The *Foundation Directory* is published by the Foundation Center and distributed by Columbia University Press. It is a directory that lists foundations alphabetically in terms of their interests and programs, program limitations, assets, officers, contact individuals, and addresses. It has three indexes: (1) areas of interest, (2) foundation names, and (3) foundation donors. The Foundation Center conducts computer searches of the directory for a modest service fee. It is located at 888 Seventh Avenue, New York, NY 10010.

The Annual Register of Grant Support is an annual publication that describes all granting agencies that allocated funds during the year previous to publication. It is published by Academic Media, 200 E. Ohio, Chicago, IL 60611.

Finally, the American Psychological Association publishes the *Guide to Research Support*. In an outline fashion this book describes all federal funding programs of interest to behavioral and social scientists. It can be obtained from the national office of the Association at 1200 Seventeenth Street, N.W., Washington, DC 20036.

Enhancing the Quality of the Application

The proposal is the document from which funding agencies will attempt to gain an understanding of the need for the proposed work, and whether the principal investigator and sponsoring institution are capable of executing the project. A well-developed proposal answers critical questions unambiguously by providing ample information and cogent justification. However, the quality of a proposal is not directly proportional to length. The following are important questions to keep in mind when structuring and writing the proposal:

1. What does the proposed project intend to do?
2. Why is the work important?
3. What has already been done?
4. How do previous studies relate to the proposed project?
5. How will the work be done?
6. Who will do the work? What are the qualifications of these people relevant to the project?
7. Where will the project be done? Is it a proposal submitted jointly by two or more institutions or organizations? What are the responsibilities and levels of accountability for each institution or organization, as well as those of individuals?
8. How much will it cost, and why?
9. How will the findings of the research be used and by whom? How will they be disseminated?
10. How will the project be evaluated and by whom?

A few of these questions are now explored in greater detail.

BIOGRAPHICAL SKETCH

The biographical sketch is the primary instrument by which reviewers evaluate the capability and ability of principal investigators and their associates to carry out the proposed research. In addition to listing educational credentials, experience, employment, and honors, it is equally important to cite previous research activity. This information should include project titles, funding sources, length of projects, and percentage of involvement. Also important is information on consultation and technical assistance provided to research projects. Publications relevant to the application should be cited, as well as all publications of the past few years.

The biographical sketch has a page limitation of two pages. It is not uncommon for applications to include the Curricula Vitae of key project personnel in the appendixes. It is preferred to focus these CVs on the proposed project and the scientific credentials of the key personnel.

CRITERIA FOR EVALUATION OF PROPOSALS

The following listing provides the dimensions along which applications for research funding are evaluated within the federal system. These are:

1. Significance of the topic (scientific, social, clinical).
2. Potential usefulness, generalizability, or heuristic value of anticipated findings.
3. Scientific merit and validity of the research plan.
4. Significance and originality of research goals.
5. Specificity of hypothesis statements.
6. Appraisal of state of knowledge in the field.
7. Completeness of literature review on proposed topic.
8. Relatedness of literature review to specific research questions and hypotheses.
9. Feasibility of the research.
10. Originality and adequacy of research methodology.
11. Appropriateness of research design.
12. Properties of instrumentation.
13. Appropriateness and detail of procedures for data analysis.
14. Indication of sample cooperation.
15. Protection of human subjects.
16. Competence and dedication of principal investigator and supporting staff.
17. Adequacy of research facility and resources.
18. Appropriateness of budget and time frame.

REASONS FOR DISAPPROVAL

In my affiliation with federal granting agencies, I have reviewed over 100 applications from nurse researchers, which have included some approvals, some deferrals, and a lot of disapprovals. Of the disapprovals, 85% showed at least one major methodological weakness. I would like to present the most common flaws, citing each one of them from my written evaluations of grant proposals:

1. "Rationale and assumptions are not clear, making the methodology inadequate."
2. "The design is fragmented and has serious defects and omissions—it will not produce the anticipated outcomes."
3. "Some methodological problems are stated but not dealt with adequately."
4. "The proposal is too vague."
5. "The proposed tests and methods are unsuited for the objectives of the proposal and the data to be collected and analyzed."
6. "Data management and processing are presented in detail, the coding schemes are elaborated; however, the scoring of the two mediating variables indirectly associated with feeding of the elderly is still unclear."
7. "The connection between the conceptualization and the execution

of the research is not clearly articulated, and the methods for testing the validity and reliability of the Confusion Inventory being developed are not described adequately."

8. "Concepts related to Orem, Rogers, and Roy models will be used. However, no specific concepts were identified; it is unclear how the concept(s) chosen from the three nursing theoretical models will relate to the final Confusion Inventory."

9. In a study of Alzheimer's Disease in four rural communities, "no reason is given for replicating the study in four communities. No definition for rural is stated. No information is included as to whether Alzheimer's Disease (AD) is a primary diagnosis or suspected. It is reported that some of the patients were diagnosed by the family whereas others were diagnosed by a family practitioner. None of them had been seen by a neurologist."

10. "While the proposal is to compare patient care outcomes when services are provided by BSN, LPN, and Diploma nurse graduates, nothing is said about the NLN competency statement, the case-mix of patients, staffing on the evening and night shifts, availability of clerical support to nursing personnel, educational levels of the head nurse and nurse supervisor, nor about staff satisfaction in general. The validity and reliability of the instruments measuring nursing care as dependent variables were not addressed."

11. In a study of depression and confusion in elderly hypertensive patients, "sample selection is questioned because many of the patients are on antihypertensive drugs that may cause depression. The onset of depression, in addition, is not adequately described."

12. In a study of the symptoms of mental illness due to Alzheimer's disease and other dementias of the oldest old (age 85+), "none of the proposed staff has extensive neuropsychological expertise or experience. It is unclear how the diagnosis of A.D. will be determined and the sample of 25 patients will be selected. The experimental designs are only sketchily outlined. Methods of analysis are not detailed."

These quotes are from my actual experience as a reviewer of applications by nurse researchers. The critiques cited are certainly not exhaustive, and additional ones have been identified over the years (Allen, 1960; Berthold, 1973; Clinton, 1985; Gortner, 1971; Lisk, 1971; Wright, 1971). Summarized, additional common reasons for disapproval are as follows:

1. Lack of new or original ideas.
2. Diffuse, superficial, or unfocused research plan.
3. Lack of knowledge of published relevant work.
4. Uncertainty concerning future directions.
5. Questionable reasoning in experimental approach.

6. Lack of sufficient experimental detail.
7. Absence of an acceptable scientific rationale.
8. Unrealistically large amount of work.
9. Uncritical approach.

Conclusion

Improving the methodological adequacy of research proposals submitted for federal funding and, consequently, enhancing the likelihood of funding for nursing research is a complex matter. Although it obviously entails issues directly pertaining to quantitative methodology and statistics, it also encompasses a myriad of other issues: conceptualization, budget, time frame, scientific credentials of the research team, and adequacy of the research environments. Efforts aimed at assisting nurse researchers in obtaining funding and at expanding the overall funding base of nursing should comprehensively integrate these different issues.

REFERENCES

Allen, E. M. (1960). Why research grant applications are disapproved. *Science, 132,* 1532–1534.
Berthold, J. S. (1973). Nursing grant proposals: What influenced their approval or disapproval in two national granting agencies. *Nursing Research, 22,* 292–299.
Clinton, J. (1985). Couvade: Patterns, predictors, and nursing management—A research proposal submitted to the Division of Nursing. *Western Journal of Nursing Research, 7,* 229–240.
Gortner, S. R. (1971). Research grant applications: What they are not and should be. *Nursing Research, 20,* 292–295.
Kehrer, B. H., Aiken, L. H., Blendon, R. J., & Rogers, D. E. (1984). The research program and priorities of the Robert Wood Johnson Foundation. *Health Services Research, 19,* 439–453.
Lisk, D. J. (1971, October 15). Why research grant applications are tuned down. *Bio Science, 21,* No. 20, October 15.
Wright, S. (1971). *Reasons for disapproval of health research project grant applications.* Internal Publications, Division of Research Grants, Research Analysis and Evaluation Branch, National Institutes of Health. Bethesda, MD: National Institutes of Health.

Comment

The Disapproval of Proposals on Methodological and Statistical Grounds

STEPHEN J. ZYZANSKI, Ph.D.

A critical section of the preceding chapter is the one that deals with the disapproval of grant applications. A variety of recurring problems extracted from the reviews of disapproved applications were cited. These included study design and methods issues, instrument reliability and validity concerns, statistical analysis and sample size problems, and issues concerning the skills and experience of the investigators, to name a few. The comments provided here highlight two of these areas: (1) issues in research design and (2) computer and statistical analysis problems.

Research Design

A major stumbling block in achieving design parity has been the failure of investigators to use properly many of the widely accepted research designs. Such designs as factorial, repeated measures, or unequal cell size are often not well understood, are misused, or simply are underutilized. Another design problem concerns the fact that little or no justification is given for including the variables to be studied. This frequently results in the gathering of too much information with no sense of priorities to help select the most important variables. A third common design problem is the often neglected subject-to-variable ratio. Designs with at least twice as many subjects as variables are far less likely to introduce statistical artifacts and produce spurious or highly biased relationships. A final design issue concerns the fact that some proposals simply do not thoroughly describe the major dependent and independent variables. Not only is this a crucial aspect of any study, but it can place reviewers at a disadvantage. Without a thorough description of the major indexes, it is extremely difficult to evaluate a proposal's potential in achieving its objectives.

Another issue related to research design pertains to confounding variables and alternative hypotheses. Investigators frequently fail to consider the various threats to the internal and external validity of their designs. All too often, the importance of other variables is not considered. Relevant control variables frequently are not included, alternative hypotheses are not considered, and thus the research findings are difficult to evaluate because too many of these factors could also have accounted for the same findings.

A third major design area is sampling issues, which includes the problem of poor or infrequent sample size estimation. Study samples can often be too big as well as too small for the purposes designed. A statistically estimated sample size saves time, effort, and often considerable expense.

A final design issue concerns the pilot study. Pilot studies potentially can play a very important role in the development of research proposals. Often this potential is not realized. Pilot studies, for example, are extremely useful for estimating sample size, testing the feasibility of the approach, assessing questionnaire length, and gaining experience with the protocol, statistical analysis, and interpretation of the results. They are helpful in training and calibrating interviewers, in assessing the usefulness of modified instruments, in deleting irrelevant variables, and, in general, in acquainting the investigator with many of the problems of conducting the study.

Statistical Analysis

Turning next to issues involved in plans and strategies of analysis, one of the glaring inadequacies encountered is the fact that all too often much of the effort is focused on collecting the data and far too little effort is directed at planning how to analyze them. Some investigators barely describe the analysis plans, providing only terse or poorly described plans. Often lists of variables are provided but no mention is made of how they are to be measured or analyzed. Too often confounding or control variables are not included in the analysis. How the variables are to be used in the analysis is an important part of any proposal.

A second analysis issue pertains to the actual application of statistical techniques, another potential source of problems. All too often inappropriate statistical tests are applied to the data. For example, the level of measurement is ignored in selecting a statistical test; tables with too many cells, either blank or with low expected values, are included in the analysis; or tests designed for independent samples are used with dependent samples. This dependency issue is particularly important for matching studies where the unit of analysis should be the pair and not the individual.

A third analysis issue is the fact that statistical assumptions are rarely checked. Too easily, data are entered into computer programs. The resulting analyses can sometimes be spurious or even meaningless, yet this is not always detected. A related problem concerns the meaning and interpretation of statistical significance. The statistical significance and clinical relevance of the data analysis are often compromised by testing too many variables while ignoring the Type I Error rates. Selecting a few presumed significant associations out of many comparisons not only is risky, but has the added problem of making sense out of many comparisons that likely include chance-level associations. Finally, it is often not realized that with small samples important results may go unrecognized, because the sample size was inadequate to detect smaller but clinically meaningful effects. This highlights the importance of the Type II Error rate, which is generally a more neglected issue than that of the Type I Error rate.

A final analysis issue concerns the increasing use of multivariate techniques. On the one hand, they offer the potential for sophisticated control of many sources of variation. On the other hand, these statistics are more difficult to compute and to interpret. Too often studies are designed as multivariate; that is, they employ multiple-outcome or dependent variables but are never analyzed as such. For example, repeated-measures designs are logically analyzed by multivariate methods, but too often they are not so analyzed. Lost from these analyses is the richness of the patterning that may be occurring across the data. Multivariate techniques can be extremely useful, but they need to be carefully thought through in planning a study, and, if possible, pilot-tested to gain experience in their use and interpretation.

Suggestions

Some suggestions for improving the quantitative aspects of research proposals might include the following. First, the scope of projects should be limited to a manageable size. The more focused the study, the more the effort can be placed on measuring a limited number of things well. Second, having relevant others (e.g., consultants) critique the proposal prior to submission is worthwhile. An independent evaluator can often identify problem areas and recommend solutions. Third, the use of the pilot study seems to be underutilized and could greatly enhance the soundness of an initial research application. Fourth, further preparation and training in research methodology also seem clearly warranted. Fifth, for a research team to be effective, a critical mass is needed, which includes at a minimum clinical expertise, research skills, and appropriate consultants. A few good consultants can often identify, in advance, many of the problems cited here and can help to design research that is fundamentally sound. Finally, a review of commonly encountered problem areas, such as the ones cited here and in the preceding chapter, is an excellent and extremely useful strategy for helping junior investigators plan and develop a grant application for funding.

14

The Presentation of Scientific Data in Nursing Research

MARGARET R. GRIER, Ph.D., F.A.A.N.
MARQUIS D. FOREMAN, Ph.D., R.N.

The scientific method is used by researchers to obtain data for testing an argument or for constructing intellectual schemata (Gore, 1981). The intent in using the scientific method is to produce data that are reliable and valid: data that are independent of personal beliefs, values, biases, attitudes, perceptions, and/or emotions (Kerlinger, 1973). The aspiration for objective data is that every individual can reach independent yet identical conclusions (Kerlinger, 1973). Such universal conclusions require not only the objective acquisition of data but also objective analysis and clear and precise description of the findings.

To present scientific data effectively, statistical methods and visual displays must be chosen to characterize clearly and economically the nature of the data in sufficient detail to justify the investigator's interpretations and conclusions (APA, 1983; Freeman, Gonzalez, Hoaglin, & Kliss, 1983; Megeath, 1975). A rigorous evaluation and description of data should prevent the uncritical acceptance of erroneous conclusions, the consequences of which can be severe (Altman, 1982). Conversely, an unclear presentation may render data uninterpretable and may indicate a lack of understanding of the findings, rationale, and analyses (Altman, 1982). Despite frequent comments (Altman, 1981, 1982; O'Fallon, Dubey, Salsburg, Edmonson, Soffer, & Colton, 1978; Reynolds & Simmonds, 1981; Schuster, Binion, Moxley, Walrath, Grassmuch, Mahnks, & Schmidt, 1976; Vaisrub, 1985) about the poor quality of the presentation of data in the scientific literature, guidelines for their presentation are absent. In this chapter, guidelines for graphic, tabular, and statistical description of data are provided. Criteria for choosing appropriate visual displays for the clear presentation of a data set are presented. Although a discussion of criteria for the selection of appropriate statistical methods is beyond the scope of this paper, recommendations for the clear presentation of those statistical procedures will be made.

Graphic Description

Graphs are a method for simultaneously organizing, summarizing, and communicating a set of data (APA, 1983; Kviz & Knafl, 1980; Megeath, 1975;

Reynolds & Simmonds, 1981). They provide less precise information than tables but are more useful for conveying an overall sense or picture of data. Graphs are best for providing a spatial representation of multiple measurements (Beniger & Robyn, 1978). Graphs are useful for demonstrating relationships, emphasizing trends, and depicting the shape of a distribution (APA, 1983; Fienberg, 1979; Jaegger, 1983; Kviz & Knafl, 1980; Megeath, 1975). Because of multiple forms, the choice of a graphic display should be based on function rather than on aesthetics (Hailstone, 1973):

1. Line graphs and diagrams are useful for depicting continuous change (APA, 1983; Schutz, 1961a, 1961b) and have been shown as best for point reading (Hailstone, 1973) and best for retention (Reynolds & Simmonds, 1981).
2. Bar charts or histograms are preferred for presenting multiple variables (Reynolds & Simmonds, 1981) and for comparing data (Hailstone, 1973).
3. Circle, or pie, graphs typically are used to show quantities, proportions, or percentages (APA, 1983; Jaegger, 1983; Reynolds & Simmonds, 1981).
4. Scatter graphs are used to depict relationships among variables (APA, 1983; Jaegger, 1983).
5. Pictorial graphs are used to represent simple quantitative differences (APA, 1983).
6. Coxcomb graphs, developed by Florence Nightingale, are useful for showing phenomena of a cyclical nature (Fienberg, 1979; Grier & Grier, 1978).

There are three rules for preparation of graphs. First, the purpose of the graph should be determined. This determination will assist in deciding the form and contents of the graph (APA, 1983; Hailstone, 1973; Reynolds & Simmonds, 1981). Second, graphic content should be intelligible independent of the text, yet provide a picture of that information. If the graph does not complement the text or more efficiently present information, the graph is not needed (APA, 1983; Gore, 1981; Reynolds & Simmonds, 1981). Third, the structure of the graph should enhance the inherent nature of the data. Findings can be enhanced by choosing between arithmetic and logarithmic grid scales, thereby intensifying the meaning of the data (APA, 1983; Campbell, 1974; Gladen & Rogan, 1983; Hailstone, 1973; Reynolds & Simmonds, 1981). However, one must be cautious that the data are not distorted (Campbell, 1974; Huff, 1954). Various graphing techniques should be used to examine the data to determine which method best represents the findings (Gore, 1981; Hailstone, 1973).

In structuring graphs, one needs to be cognizant not only of how a graph affects the picture of findings, but also of how human information processing is impacted by the graph (Tinker, 1965). Individuals become increasingly confused and less able to obtain meaning from graphs as the lines exceed four (Schutz, 1961a, 1961b). The goal of any visual display is to depict and summarize findings by eliminating redundancy without losing vital information (Hailstone, 1973; Jaegger, 1983). Consequently, graphs should be simple; they should contain no more than four lines or curves; and geometrical forms should be plain and distinct (APA, 1983; Hailstone, 1973; Reynolds & Simmonds, 1981).

In brief, graphs are an efficient method of presenting information when the purpose is to demonstrate relationships visually in a set of data. Graphs provide a picture and overview and are useful for building a cognitive framework for placing subsequent detailed data to support conclusions.

Tabular Description

Tables are an array or matrix of numbers with certain characteristics or categories and are useful for simultaneously and concisely organizing, summarizing, and communicating a set of precise data (APA, 1983; Knapp, 1978; Kviz & Knafl, 1980; Megeath, 1975). Tables are recommended for presenting the exact data on which an inference is based (Megeath, 1975). Because of their construction and composition, tabular displays permit a parsimonious description of more complete data than what can be presented in text form. Unless properly constructed, however, tabular displays of data can be difficult to interpret and understand.

Rules to guide the preparation of tables parallel those for graphs. First, determine precisely the purpose of a table. If the audience needs precise numerical data rapidly and accurately, a tabular presentation is the best choice (Carter, 1947; Reynolds & Simmonds, 1981). The specific content of a table is best determined by asking three questions (APA, 1983; Megeath, 1975; Reynolds & Simmonds, 1981):

1. What relationships and trends need to be demonstrated?
2. What information does the reader already have and what additional information should be gained from the table?
3. How many additional data are needed for comprehension of the information in the text?

Answers to these questions will assist in determining whether the table should consist of exact values or rounded-off values (APA, 1983). Rounded values are more easily understood and remembered. Decimal values, usually not exceeding two places, should be used only when necessary to ascertain the results and when appropriate to the variables being described.

Second, tabular contents should be intelligible independent of the text, and not repeat information discussed in the text (APA, 1983; Megeath, 1975;

Reynolds & Simmonds, 1981). Tables also should present information explicitly (Carter, 1947; Reynolds & Simmonds, 1981; Wright & Fox, 1970). For instance, computations necessary for comprehending the findings should be included in the table. Explicit tables require less effort on the part of the reader and lessen the chances for confusion and misinterpretation from computational errors (Carter, 1947; Reynolds & Simmonds, 1981; Wright & Fox, 1970).

Third, the structure of a table should convey the information in a way that is compatible with human information processing (APA, 1983; Reynolds & Simmonds, 1981; Woodward, 1972). Western cultures use a left-to-right and top-to-bottom strategy for processing information. Therefore, the following four guidelines are recommended to facilitate the communication of tabular information:

1. Construct tables according to their function. Tables in which numbers are to be compared should be constructed of columns rather than rows, since it is easier to compare numerical data from left to right than to compare them up and down (APA, 1983; Reynold & Simmonds, 1981; Tinker, 1965). Conversely, the comparison of verbal material is best in rows (Frase, 1969); words are compared more easily in a vertical format than in a horizontal format.

2. Data should be grouped within a table according to their demonstrated relationships, since items in close physical proximity are perceived as closely related (Reynolds & Simmonds, 1981). Columnar groupings of five items are most effective in conveying information (Tinker, 1965).

3. Spacing between columns and rows also facilitates the scanning of information. Horizontal scanning is enhanced when spacing is greater between rows, whereas vertical scanning is enhanced when spacing is greater between columns (APA, 1983; Reynolds & Simmonds, 1981).

4. Headings should logically describe and organize the data within a table, with definitions and additional information in footnotes when necessary (APA, 1983; Reynolds & Simmonds). Information in the table heading should not repeat the row and column headings. Headings to the table, rows and columns, should correspond to information that the reader already possesses and should provide direction for seeking information from the table (Reynolds & Simmonds, 1981).

In summary, tables, if properly constructed, are a concise and effective means for organizing, summarizing, and communicating a set of data. The purpose of data in tables is to convey a more complete set of precise values more rapidly and accurately than can be communicated through text and graphs. The construction of tables should facilitate the reader's comprehension of the information the investigator wishes to convey with this mode of communication.

Statistical Description

Statistics are an even more concise way to communicate findings than are verbal, graphic, or tabular descriptions. Prior to the 1600s and the development of scientific instrumentation, data were hand collected and reported in their raw form. But the continued growth in scientific instrumentation led to such increased quantities of data that they could no longer be presented in their totality. Thus, the science of statistics, a fundamental component of the scientific method (Hooke, 1980), developed to handle the collection, organization, analysis, interpretation, and communication of masses of numerical data. Within half a line of print, the phrase $F(2,120) = 10.47$, $p < .001$ says what statistical procedure was used to evaluate the data, the comparison, the statistical value for the comparison, and the likelihood of observing the difference by chance. Moreover, all this is said in a form that is verifiable.

Statistical methods enable a researcher logically and rationally to screen, evaluate, integrate, and communicate data meaningfully (Garvey, 1979). Yet many believe statistics in the biomedical literature are misused and that they communicate distorted or erroneous information (Altman, 1981, 1982; Beattie, Donovan, Mant, & Bridges-Webb, 1984; Campbell, 1974; Finney, 1982; Glantz, 1980; Hooke, 1980, 1983; Huff, 1954; O'Fallon et al., 1978; Schor & Karten, 1966; Schuster et al., 1976; Stempel, 1982; Vaisrub, 1985). Critical reviews of the British and American biomedical literature consistently found errors in 50% of those studies using statistical procedures (Altman, 1981; Glantz, 1980; Schor & Karten, 1966; Vaisrub, 1985). The most frequently occurring statistical errors were inappropriate research designs for the stated problem; inappropriate statistical procedures for the questions or data; calculations that are improperly and incompetently performed; and interpretations that are incorrect or extrapolated beyond the limits of the data (Altman, 1982; Finney, 1982; Glantz, 1980; O'Fallon et al., 1978; Schor & Karten, 1966). Errors and misinterpretations also result from lifting data directly from computer print-out sheets (Altman, 1982; Glantz, 1980)—for example, inappropriate use of uppercase letters, to which some machines are restricted (P for p), and reporting p values of .0000 when such values must be greater than zero.

The misuse of statistical methods is a serious ethical and scientific issue with consequences potentially harmful to subjects and to the scientific community. Statistical errors can result in the unwarranted exposure of subjects to risks and inconvenience, and the needless consumption of scarce research resources (Altman, 1982; Glantz, 1980). If uncritically accepted, unreliable results can influence and mislead other scientific investigators (Altman, 1982; Glantz, 1980), a problem exacerbated by failing to provide readers with sufficient information to evaluate the results and associated interpretations adequately (Glantz, 1980).

In response to the misuse of statistics, the following four recommendations are offered (Altman, 1981, 1982; APA, 1983; Finney, 1982; Freeman et al., 1983; Glantz, 1980; Hooke, 1980; O'Fallon et al., 1978; Vaisrub, 1985):

1. The research team should include a statistician as an integral member, or statistical consultation should be sought throughout all phases of the research.
2. The approval of a research proposal by the ethical review board should include an evaluation of the proposed statistical analysis, with approval based on appropriateness and correctness of the proposed analysis.
3. The review of all manuscripts submitted for publication in scientific journals should include a statistical review by an experienced statistician.
4. The report of statistical analysis should clearly describe and justify all procedures used; demonstrate that all assumptions for the use of those statistical procedures were met; present only those data relevant to the questions asked; provide a measure of the variability in the observations; provide quantitative results (means and standard deviations) in addition to significance levels; and distinguish between statistical and clinical significance.

The development of universal standards for the content and format of statistical data in manuscripts has been recommended (O'Fallon et al., 1978). The American Psychological Association (APA) provided guidelines for reporting inferential statistics. In the APA (1983) *Publication Manual* investigators are instructed to provide the symbol of the statistic, the degrees of freedom, the magnitude or value of the test, and the probability level, as well as the mean, standard deviation, or other descriptive statistics to show the nature of the effect. Such content should be included whether the statistic is reported by text, graph, or table.

Proper statistical statements are the most concise and precise way to report the results of data analysis. Statistical techniques are a means to screen, evaluate, integrate, and communicate the findings from large amounts of data in a logical way (Garvey, 1979). Care must be taken, however, that all the necessary information is included within a statistical phrase.

Summary

Specific guidelines for the presentation of scientific data are presented in the appendix to this paper (p. 197). Investigators should ascertain what conclusions should be reported and how best to describe the data supporting that conclusion. The data should be presented in a clear, concise, logical, and precise manner, as well as in a way that facilitates comprehension and retention by the reader. The reader should be provided a picture of the findings through graphical displays, followed by more complete and precise arrays of data in a table. Once the reader has a picture of the results in mind and a precise and complete set of data in hand, a statistical phrase that concisely describes the evaluation of the findings should be presented. The benefits of adhering to these guidelines for the presentation of scientific data are a decrease in untoward consequences to research subjects, the wise use of research resources, the effective communication of vital information, and the advancement of science and nursing.

REFERENCES

Altman, D. G. (1981). Statistics and ethics in medical research. VIII—Improving the quality of statistics in medical journals. *British Medical Journal 282*, 44–47.

Altman, D. G. (1982). Statistics in medical journals. *Statistics in Medicine, 1,* 59–71.

American Psychological Association. (1983). *The publication manual of the American Psychological Association* (3rd ed.). Washington, DC: The Association.

Beattie, A., Donovan, B., Mant, A., & Bridges-Webb, C. (1984). Interpretation and presentation of results: Chickens will come home to roost. *Australian Family Physician, 13,* 429–430.

Beniger, J. R., & Robyn, D. L. (1978). Quantitative graphics in statistics: A brief history. *The American Statistician, 32,* 1–11.

Campbell, S. K. (1974). *Flaws and fallacies in statistical thinking.* Englewood Cliffs, NJ: Prentice-Hall.

Carter, L. F. (1947). An experiment on the design of tables and graphs used for presenting numerical data. *Journal of Applied Psychology, 31,* 640–650.

Fienberg, S. E. (1979). Graphical methods in statistics. *The American Statistician, 33,* 165–178.

Finney, D. J. (1982). The questioning statistician. *Statistics in Medicine, 1,* 5–13.

Frase, L. T. (1969). Tabular and diagrammatic presentation of verbal materials. *Perceptual and Motor Skills, 29,* 320–322.

Freeman, D. H., Jr., Gonzalez, M. E., Hoaglin, D. C., & Kliss, B. A. (1983). Presenting statistical papers. *The American Statistician, 37,* 106–110.

Garvey, W. D. (1979). *Communication: The essence of science.* Oxford: Pergamon.

Gladen, B. C., & Rogan, W. J. (1983). On graphing rate ratios. *American Journal of Epidemiology, 118,* 905–908.

Glantz, S. A. (1980). Biostatistics: How to detect, correct, and prevent errors in the medical literature. *Circulation, 61,* 1–7.

Gore, S. M. C. (1981). Assessing methods—Descriptive statistics and graphs. *British Medical Journal, 283,* 486–488.

Grier, B., & Grier, M. (1978). Contributions of the passionate statistician. *Research in Nursing and Health, 1,* 103–109.

Hailstone, M. (1973). A case for standardization in the preparation of graphs and diagrams. *Medical and Biological Illustrations, 23,* 8–12.

Hooke, R. (1980). Getting people to use statistics properly. *The American Statistician, 34,* 39–42.

Hooke, R. (1983). *How to tell liars from the statisticians.* New York: Marcel Dekker.

Huff, D. (1954). *How to lie with statistics.* New York: Norton.

Jaegger, R. M. (1983). *Statistics: A spectator sport.* Beverly Hills, CA: Sage.

Kerlinger, F. N. (1973). *Foundations of behavioral research* (2nd ed.). New York: Holt.

Knapp, R. G. (1978). *Basic statistics for nurses.* New York: Wiley.

Kviz, F. J., & Knafl, K. A. (1980). *Statistics for nurses: An introductory text.* Boston: Little, Brown.

Megeath, J. D. (1975). *How to use statistics.* New York: Canfield.

O'Fallon, J. R., Dubey, S. D., Salsburg, D. S., Edmonson, J. H., Soffer, A., & Colton, T. (1978). Should there be statistical guidelines for medical research papers? *Biometrics, 34,* 687–695.

Reynolds, L., & Simmonds, D. (1981). *Presentation of data in science.* The Hague: Martinus-Nijhoff.

Schor, S., & Karten, I. (1966). Statistical evaluation of medical journal manuscripts. *Journal of the American Medical Association, 195,* 145–150.

Schuster, J. J., Binion, J., Moxley, J., Walrath, N., Grassmuch, D., Mahnks, D., & Schmidt, J. (1976). Recommended procedures for biomedical research articles (editorial). *Journal of the American Medical Association, 235,* 534–535.

Schutz, H. G. (1961a). An evaluation of formats for graphic trend display—Experiment II. *Human Factors, 3,* 99–107.

Schutz, H. G. (1961b). An evaluation of methods for presentation of graphic multiple trends—Experiment III. *Human Factors, 3,* 108–119.

Stempel, L. E. (1982). Eenie, meenie, minie, mo... What do the data really show. *American Journal of Obstetrics and Gynecology, 144,* 745–752.

Tinker, M. A. (1965). *Bases for effective reading.* Minneapolis: University of Minnesota Press.

Vaisrub, N. (1985). Manuscript review from a statistician's perspective (editorial). *Journal of the American Medical Association, 253,* 3145–3147.

Woodward, R. M., Jr. (1972). Proximity and direction of arrangement in numerical displays. *Human Factors, 14,* 337–343.

Wright, P., & Fox, K. (1970). Presenting information in tables. *Applied Ergonomics, 1,* 234–242.

APPENDIX
GUIDELINES FOR THE PRESENTATION OF SCIENTIFIC DATA

I. Determine precisely what is to be communicated and select only the material that will convey relevant information about the topic.
  A. What questions and/or issues will be raised from the conclusion that will need to be explained and/or supported by the data?
  B. What relationships and trends in the data will need to be demonstrated?
  C. What information will the audience have prior to the presentation of the data?
  D. What additional information should be gained from the data?
  E. How much additional information will be required to comprehend the findings?
II. Choose the medium—graphs, tables, statistics—that best present the data clearly and concisely:
  A. Graphic displays provide an overview of findings and are useful for building a cognitive framework for placing subsequent detailed data. In constructing graphs:
    1. Examine the data using various graphic forms; choose the form that most accurately and appropriately conveys the nature of the findings.
    2. Choose the grid scale (arithmetic or logarithmic) that best intensifies the information from the data, taking care that the selected scale does not distort the data and is correctly proportioned.
    3. Plot the data accurately.
    4. Construct the graph so that it
      a. is intelligible and independent of the text.
      b. complements or more efficiently presents information.
      c. summarizes the data.
      d. eliminates redundancy without omitting information.
      e. contains no more than four lines or curves.
      f. contains geometric forms that are plain and distinct.
    5. Spell all terms correctly and explain all abbreviations and symbols in a legend or the caption.
    6. Use all symbols, abbreviations, and terminology in the graph consistently as compared with those in the caption, legend, other graphs, and text.
  B. Tabular displays provide precise numerical information rapidly and accurately. When constructing tables,
    1. Use titles to provide a concise explanation of the information in the table.
    2. Use column and row headings that correspond to the information previously provided and that direct attention to the additional information provided by the table.
    3. Construct the table so that it
      a. is intelligible and independent of the text.
      b. does not repeat information discussed in the text.
      c. demonstrates differences and similarities in the data.
      d. facilitates the scanning of information through the use of organization and spacing.
      e. presents information explicitly.
    4. Explain all abbreviations, underlines, parentheses, and special symbols.
    5. Correctly report all probability levels. The correct symbol should be used to denote the probability level, and asterisks should be attached to the appropriate table entries.
  C. Statistical methods enable a researcher to screen, evaluate, and integrate relevant information logically as well as to communicate it meaningfully and concisely.
    1. Present only those data relevant to the questions asked.
    2. Provide sufficient information for evaluating the adequacy and appropriateness of all analytic methods used and their associated interpretations and conclusions.
    3. Report the symbol of the statistic, the associated degrees of freedom, the magnitude or value of the test, the probability level, as well as the mean, standard deviation, or other descriptive statistic of the effect.
    4. Distinguish between statistical and clinical significance.

Comment

The Presentation of Scientific Data in Context

MARY ANN PRICE SWAIN, Ph.D.

The previous chapter is written at two levels of discourse. First, it is a straightforward presentation of guidelines for developing tables and graphs. A substantial amount of information is culled from a variety of sources and is nicely pulled together and organized. The discussion on choice of graphic display for presenting particular kinds of information (e.g., the use of line graphs for depicting continuous change and the use of pie graphs for showing proportions) is instructive. Nevertheless, the rules for preparation of graphs and tables are fairly abstract, and it is unclear whether they are sufficient to instruct someone to become adept at using graphic displays. The observations on limits and tendencies in human information processing were also helpful. Only so much information can be gleaned from a single table or graph and the degree of visual clarity can improve understanding. Furthermore, our Western cultural tendencies to read from left to right and from top to bottom do have an impact on one's ability to comprehend information in tables. Calling this matter to the attention of an investigator adds an important dimension to thinking about developing a graphic or tabular display.

Although the proposed guidelines for the reporting of statistical analyses do not raise any concerns, discussion preceding their delineation is at a different (and second) level of discourse.

At that point the chapter no longer focuses merely on the presentation of scientific data but becomes a critique of the entire methodological plan for the collection, analysis, and interpretation of data. One could disagree with the definition of statistical errors as including inappropriate research designs for the stated problem and unjustified interpretations of the data. These are errors but not statistical ones. The use of statistics is only one aspect of the conduct of science; it is not the entire scientific method. Statistical errors do legitimately include, as stated, inappropriate statistical procedures for the questions or data and calculations that are improperly or incompletely performed.

Certainly, poorly conceived research can result in what was described as the unwanted exposure of subjects to risk and inconvenience and the needless consumption of scarce resources, because faulty designs render the data virtually useless. Thus, ethical review boards should look at the appropriateness of the entire research design for answering the question raised or addressing the problem presented. But any critique of the selection of the statistical method must be considered in the light of the relationship of the entire data collection process to the questions themselves. Reviewers have often collapsed a critical evaluation of a completed project into assessing the preceding statistical approach when, in fact, the statistical approach was entirely justified, given the level of measurements used, the shape of the distribution of obtained values, and the number of cases present. The more fundamental error tends to occur not in the statistics but in the gross mismatch between the theoretical concepts themselves and their operationalization in the measures selected. Thus, perhaps not the statistical validity of the project should be questioned, but the extent to which it has bearing on the theory that directed it.

Another issue related to the preceding chapter has to do with assumptions underlying the section on statistical errors, which may create the impression that there is no disagreement among statisticians about how to analyze data. The suggestions that every research team should include a statistician as an integral member and that no manuscript should be passed without the review of an experienced statistician imply that all statisticians would agree on how to handle a particular data set. The continuing controversy over the treatment of ordinal data is a good example of the extent to which experts disagree (Adams, Fagot, & Robinson, 1965; Gardner, 1975; Labovitz, 1972; Maxwell & Delaney, 1985; O'Brien, 1979; Wilson, 1971). For some statisticians the use of the Pearson's r

presumes that the measures employed are intervally scaled (Senders, 1958; Siegel, 1956; Townsend & Ashby, 1984). Others argue that this parametric statistic may be used with ordinal data (Baggaley & Hull, 1983; Baker, Hardyck, & Petrinovich, 1966; Borgatta, 1968; Labovitz, 1970). Thus, whether or not there is an error in choice of statistical technique, given the level of measurement, depends upon one's judgments regarding the persuasiveness of these opposing arguments. It is not that it is wrong to suggest seeking the input of a statistician, but no single recommendation is necessarily definitive.

Casting the entire discussion in terms of statistical errors presumes a primacy of Type I Errors over Type II Errors. The relationship between theory and research is conceptualized as the degree of fit or misfit between interrelationships of abstract, latent constructs and observed patterns among measured variables. In trying to bring the theoretical and empirical worlds together there are two ways to be right and two ways to be wrong. But within this decision context, statistical significance is nothing more than a conditional probability; as Hays (1963) noted, "one has observed something relatively unlikely given the hypothetical situation, but relatively more likely given some alternative situation" (p. 299). Statistical significance should not dictate either theoretical or practice decisions. What one decides based upon that information must take into account the possible losses and costs of being wrong. Concern with alpha errors is certainly warranted in situations where the experimental nursing intervention has potentially harmful side effects. One would want to be very certain that the beneficial outcomes of the intervention were not attributed to chance. But if the experimental nursing intervention were at least as effective and as safe as current practice and potentially even better, Type II Errors would become the more costly.

False prophecy is indeed a real concern to the scientific community. Scientific advancement depends upon the quality of the ideas as well as the dedication of spirit to pursue and pay serious attention to empirical data. One does not grow a strong plant from sterile seeds, but a good idea is to be nurtured carefully before one can expect the shoots to spring up. A waste of scarce resources also occurs when an investigator abandons what is actually the right way to go.

Part of the problem, particularly for the behavioral sciences, that results in directing so much attention to alpha errors stems from the relative lack of a strong tradition of replication in these sciences. Investigators do not repeat the same experiments over and over in order to increase confidence in the relationship demonstrated. Therefore, single projects take on a level of importance that is probably never justified. What we really need is an equal emphasis on the importance of theory and the sophistication of statistical techniques and a strong commitment to replication and serial projects that build one upon another. This is the best avenue to advancing nursing science and practice.

REFERENCES

Adams, E. W., Fagot, R. F., & Robinson, R. E. (1965). A theory of appropriate statistics. *Psychometrics, 30*, 99–127.

Baggaley, A. R. & Hull, A. L. (1983). The effect of nonlinear transformations on a Likert scale. *Evaluation and the Health Professions, 6*, 483–491.

Baker, B. O., Hardyck, C. D., & Petrinovich, L. F. (1966). Weak measurements vs. strong statistics: An empirical critique of S.S. Stevens' proscriptions on statistics. *Educational and Psychological Measurement, 26*, 291–309.

Borgatta, E. F. (1968). My student, the purist: A Lament. *Sociological Quarterly, 9*, 29–34.

Gardner, P. L. (1975). Scales and statistics. *Review of Educational Research, 45*, 43–57.

Hays, W. L. (1963). *Statistics*. New York: Holt.

Labovitz, S. (1970). The assignment of numbers to rank order categories. *American Sociological Review, 35*, 515–524.

Labovitz, S. (1972). Statistical usage in sociology: Sacred cows and ritual. *Sociological Methods and Research, 1*, 13–37.

Maxwell, S. E., & Delaney, H. D. (1985). Measurement and statistics: An examination of construct validity. *Psychological Bulletin, 97*, 85–93.

O'Brien, R.M. (1979). The use of Pearson's *r* with ordinal data. *American Sociological Review, 44*, 851–857.

Senders, V. L. (1958). *Measurement and statistics*. New York: Oxford.

Siegel, S. (1956). *Nonparametric statistics for the behavioral sciences*, Vol. 5. New York: Wiley.

Townsend, J. C., & Ashby, F. G. (1984). Measurement scales and statistics: The misconception misconceived. *Psychological Bulletin, 96*, 394–401.

Wilson, T. P. (1971). Critique of ordinal variables. *Social Forces, 49*, 432–444.

15

Issues and Imperatives in Instrumentation in Nursing Research

CAROLYN F. WALTZ, Ph.D., R.N.
ORA L. STRICKLAND, Ph.D., F.A.A.N.

The development of adequate, sophisticated, and methodologically rigorous methods of measuring the work of nursing programs and activities in
clinical and educational settings is a salient concern for nurses who are engaged or interested in researching the relationship between nursing processes
and outcomes. Pressures both internal and external to the nursing profession
resulting from decreased economic and manpower resources and from political forces have contributed to increased nursing interest and, one would expect, activity in this regard. In a profession like nursing in which the results of
such measurements are likely to be applied to the solution of significant
problems across educational or practice settings, the employment of sound
measurement principles and practices, especially as they are related to reliability and validity, become of utmost importance.

The purpose of this chapter is to (1) examine the measurement practices of nurse researchers undertaking studies of processes and outcomes
published in the 1984 literature and (2) from this examination of the literature, identify issues and imperatives in the measurement of process and
outcome variables reflected in these practices that warrant attention by
nurses if the reliability and validity of such studies are to be assured.

State of the Art of Nursing Process
and Outcome Measurement in 1984

As part of a larger study to assess the measurement of research variables in nursing, we used a content analysis procedure to assess process

and outcome studies appearing in 1984 in three nursing journals that were most cited by core nursing journals from 1981 to 1983 (Garfield, 1984): *Nursing Research, International Journal of Nursing Studies,* and *Research in Nursing and Health.* It is our view that, since articles published in these journals were subjected to peer review, their contents could serve as a barometer of what nurses are doing in the area of measurement, as well as what is believed to be important for sharing regarding the measurement properties of tools with other members of the profession. Only those articles that provided original qualitative or quantitative research findings that described research procedures and instrumentation within the text of the article were included. Consequently, research reviews and theoretical papers that were not presented as original research investigations were excluded from the analysis.

We developed a content analysis form that was designed to (1) specify characteristics of published nursing research studies that utilized measurement tools; (2) delineate the reported application of measurement principles and practices; (3) identify research variables studied; and (4) identify the characteristics and metric properties of measurement tools based on information provided in the articles. Items on the content analysis form and criteria for assessment of articles were generated based on content, principles, and practices propagated by measurement textbooks (Martuza, 1977; Nunnally, 1978; Waltz, Strickland, & Lenz, 1984). The content analysis form was submitted to two content specialists who held doctorates and who had preparation and experience in measurement and nursing research. A content validity index of 1.00 was obtained based on the experts' ratings of items on the tool. The interrater reliability of the tool was assessed by random selection of five articles for content analysis by two raters. An interrater reliability of .92 determined by percent agreement between raters was obtained. As the content analysis form generated descriptive data, we report our findings in terms of frequencies and percentages.

Process was defined as the manner or approach by which a program or provider delivers services to clients; outcomes were the topics or results of the program or the activities of the provider (Waltz, Strickland, & Lenz, 1984). A total of 99 articles was published during this time period that met the criteria for inclusion in the study, and 75 of these were oriented toward the study of nursing processes or outcomes. More specifically, of the 75, 28% focused on the assessment of processes, 24% on outcomes, and 48% examined the relationship between processes and outcomes. Thus, at first glance, it appears that the salience of this topic is accompanied by increased activity directed toward the measurement of processes, outcomes, and their interrelationships. Upon closer scrutiny, however, the majority of the 48% of the studies examining the relationships between processes and outcomes were found to be problematic to analyze. This resulted primarily from the fact that in many instances both the process and outcome variables were operationalized using the same tool and that descriptions of the work were such that it was difficult at best to ascertain what variables were viewed as process and what as outcomes within the context of the study, especially in the absence of an apparent link between the conceptualization and operationalization of the variables. For this reason attention here is given only to the studies focused solely on processes or outcomes ($n = 39$).

A total of 101 variables was examined in the 39 studies that focused solely on processes or outcomes; 43 were process variables and 58 were outcome variables. Of the 43 process variables, 37 (86%) were measured using only one tool or method, which, moreover, usually was developed by the researcher for the current study. The same was true for 48 (83%) of the 58 outcome variables. That is, a total of 17 process-oriented and five outcome-oriented tools was employed for the measurement of 85 variables. Thus, it appears that, although activities directed toward studying processes and outcomes represent a high proportion of the nursing research published in 1984, activities within the context of these studies directed toward measurement of process and outcome variables were actually quite limited.

To determine further the measurement practices of nurses undertaking the study of processes and outcomes, the 22 tools and methods employed for the measurement of these 85 variables were scrutinized to ascertain (1) the primary focus of the work, (2) the conceptual basis underlying the tool's or method's development, and (3) measurement practices employed.

PRIMARY FOCUS OF THE WORK

The primary focus of the work was categorized using categories based on criteria adapted from Gortner, Bloch, and Phillips (1976) and Bloch (1981) for classifying nursing questions into four areas of nursing research: nursing care, nursing services delivery, nursing education, and research on the profession of nursing. The fifth category, development of research methods or tools, was added by the authors. The data are summarized in Table 15–1.

Results indicated that the primary focus of the work in the case of both processes and outcomes was nursing care research, with the highest proportion of process studies addressing fundamental as opposed to applied

TABLE 15–1. PRIMARY FOCUS OF WORK BY ORIENTATION OF STUDY				
	Process Study (n = 17)		Outcome Study (n = 5)	
Primary Focus of Work	Frequency	%	Frequency	%
Nursing care	12	71	3	60
Fundamental	9	53	1	20
Applied	3	18	2	40
Nursing education	2	12	0	0
Nursing service delivery	2	12	1	20
Research on profession	0	0	1	20
Development of research methods or tools	1	6	0	0

research. Emphasis on nursing education was minimal in the process studies (12%) and nonexistent in the outcome studies. Development of research methods or tools was the primary focus in only one process article and not at all in outcome articles.

To ascertain the nature of the specific variables selected for study, the 85 variables were listed and categorized to ascertain whether they were clinical or nonclinical in nature and, in the case of clinical variables, whether they addressed clients or nurses and health care providers. As would be expected on the basis of the primary focus of the work, in both cases variables selected for study were most often clinical in nature and focused on clients rather than on nurses and other health care providers. This suggests that in most cases the variables selected for study were consistent with the study focus. In addition, process variables, as noted by Bloch (1975), tended to focus either on services or care received by the clients or on services or care provided by the nurse; whereas outcome variables suggested by Donabedian (1970) focused upon a variety of client states and behaviors, such as level of satisfaction with care, knowledge of illness, and compliance with prescribed health regimen.

The variables measured were largely attitudinal or perceptual in the case of process variables (76%); outcome variables tended to be either behavioral/performance (40%) or record-oriented (40%). In both instances, the majority of the tools or methods employed were quantitative and utilized multiple indicators of the variables measured.

CONCEPTUAL BASIS UNDERLYING THE TOOL'S DEVELOPMENT

A conceptual framework for the tool's development was not identified in 100% of the outcome studies and 65% of the process studies. This finding raises concern regarding the appropriateness of the variables selected for study. That is, when nurses' measurement concerns emanate from an empirical rather than a conceptual point of view, there is a higher probability of investigating and measuring these variables from a more esoteric or limited perspective that overlooks important variable dimensions to be measured. During the measurement of processes and outcomes the specification of a conceptual framework is of particular importance. Since most processes are not unitary phenomena, the specific process that is the focus of measurement must be defined via the explication of a conceptual framework that captures the essence of its characteristics and identifies key variables of the process, as well as key relationships between variables. As with process measurement, no single concept is likely to be the only outcome of the particular intervention or process. Hence, the outcome variables selected for measurement must be based on and be consistent with the conceptual framework of the process or intervention that is believed to be antecedent to them. Of the six process studies in which a conceptual

TABLE 15–2. FORMAT AND APPROACH OF PROCESS
AND OUTCOME TOOLS AND METHODS

Format of Tool or Method	Process (n = 17)		Outcome (n = 5)	
	Frequency	%	Frequency	%
Multiple choice	3	18	0	0
Rating scale	1	6	2	40
Checklist	0	0	0	0
Interview—face to face	6	35	1	20
Interview—phone	1	6	0	0
Survey	5	29	0	0
Questionnaire	9	53	0	0
Record review	0	0	3	60
Semantic differential	1	6	0	0
Short answer	2	12	0	0
Vignettes	2	12	1	20
Categorization of phenomenon on basis of specified criterion	1	6	1	20
Physical measure	1	6	0	0
Approach to data collection				
Direct observation	2	12	0	0
Indirect observation	0	0	2	40
Self-report	14	82	1	20
Content analysis	1	6	2	40
Objective instrumentation	1	6	0	0

framework was employed, five had tools with framework and purposes that were consistent with the conceptual framework utilized.

An identifiable measurement framework was employed for the majority of the process tools (83%) but not for the outcome tools (40%). Process tools were more apt to be criterion referenced than to be either norm referenced or a combination of both. Given the proportion of outcome variables that were behavioral or performance oriented, it was disappointing to find that only one was developed using a criterion-referenced measurement framework.

MEASUREMENT PRACTICES

As stated earlier, most of the process tools measured care, as well as client-focused attitudinal or perceptual variables, using multiple indicators and quantitative methods. In contrast, outcome tools tended to measure nursing care, client- and provider-focused behavioral–performance variables or record-type variables, again using multiple indicators and quantitative methods. The specific format and approaches used by the tools are presented in Table 15–2. It is evident from this table that various formats were employed by each type of measure, which is not surprising, given the emphasis on the employment of multiple indicators of a variable. Also, in light of the attitudinal focus, process tools most often were questionnaires, interviews, or surveys that used a self-report approach and therefore were likely to yield quantitative data.

TABLE 15–3. RELIABILITY AND VALIDITY PRACTICES IN
REGARD TO PROCESS AND OUTCOME MEASUREMENT

Type of Reliability Data Provided	Process (n = 17)		Outcome (n = 5)	
	Frequency	%	Frequency	%
None	13	76	3	60
Test–Retest	1	6	1	20
Internal consistency	1	6	0	0
Interrater	2	12	1	20
Source of Reliability Data				
Obtained by researchers in				
context of current study	4	24	2	40
Obtained by others in previous work	0	0	0	0
Type of Validity Data Provided				
None	6	35	3	60
Face validity	4	24	1	20
Content validity	9	53	1	20
Construct	1	6	1	20
Criterion-related validity	1	6	1	20
Source of Validity Data				
Obtained by researchers in				
context of current study	11	65	2	40
Obtained by others in previous work	0	0	0	0

Outcome tools, on the other hand, relied heavily on record review as well as rating scales that used content analysis and indirect observational approaches for data collection. This finding raises concern for two reasons. First, behavioral–performance variables, which were the focus of 40% of the outcome tools, are best measured using direct observation; second, a myriad of well-documented reliability and validity problems occur with the use of record review as a sole source of data. For example, the purposes, circumstances, and procedures by which records were initially compiled greatly influence the validity of measurements based on them and obtained via content analysis.

Results with regard to reliability and validity practices in process and outcome measurement were the most disappointing in this study. As can be seen from Table 15–3, in 76% of the process studies and 60% of the outcome studies no reliability data regarding the tools were provided. If reliability estimates were available, they tended to have been obtained by the researcher within the context of the current work. Further, these reliability data were obtained utilizing only one approach, which most often was relatively simple and/or conveniently obtained (e.g., interrater, test–retest, or internal consistency reliability).

Validity data were provided in 65% of the process studies but in only 40% of the outcome studies. The higher proportion of process studies providing validity data (65%) relative to the proportion providing evidence for reliability (27%) suggests that researchers may have violated a basic tenet of measurement that reliability is a necessary but not sufficient prerequisite to validity. The validity data obtained in process studies were collected within the context of the current work and tended to provide evidence for content validity. Among outcome studies that reported validity data, it was positive to note that 40% of these used more than one approach, including content, construct, and criterion-related validity. In process studies (24%) and outcome studies (20%), researchers reported evidence for face validity. Yet this is not generally accepted as a form of validity per se; rather, it is viewed as a strategy for motivating respondents by having the tool appear to subjects to measure what they are told it measures.

SUMMARY OF FINDINGS

Findings from this review of the 1984 literature on process and outcome studies in nursing suggested that:

1. Although activities directed toward studying processes and outcomes represent a high proportion of the nursing research published in 1984, activities within the context of these studies directed toward measurement of process and outcome variables were actually quite limited, as evidenced by the measurement of 85 variables using only 22 tools.
2. The primary focus of the work in both process and outcome studies was nursing care research, with the highest proportion of process studies addressing fundamental research. Emphasis on research in nursing education was minimal in the process studies (12%) and nonexistent in the outcome studies. Development of research methods or tools was the primary focus of the work undertaken in only one process article.
3. In both process and outcome studies, variables selected were primarily clinical and focused more often on clients than on nurses and other health care providers. In most cases variables selected for study were consistent with the study focus.
4. The variables measured were largely attitudinal or perceptual in the case of process variables (76%); outcome variables tended to be behavioral–performance (40%) or record oriented (40%).
5. In both cases, the majority of the tools or methods employed were quantitative and utilized multiple indicators of the variables measured.
6. Conceptual frameworks were not cited for the tool's development in 100% of the outcome studies and 65% of the process studies.
7. In five of the six process studies (83%) in which a conceptual framework was employed, the resulting tool's framework and purposes were consistent with the conceptual framework utilized.
8. An identifiable measurement framework was employed for the majority of the process tools (83%) and the framework most often employed was criterion referenced. Only 40% of the outcome tools were developed using a measurement framework, and the

framework was criterion referenced in 20% of the cases and norm referenced in the other 20%.

9. A variety of tool formats were employed in both process and outcome studies. Appropriately, in light of the attitudinal focus, process tools most often were questionnaires, interviews, or surveys that used a self-report approach to data collection and such methods as multiple choice likely to yield quantitative data. Outcome tools relied heavily on record reviews and rating scales using content analysis and indirect observational approaches to data collection.

10. In 76% of the process studies and 60% of the outcome studies, no reliability data regarding the tools were provided. In the few cases in which reliability data were provided, they were obtained by the researcher within the context of the current work but usually involved only one relatively simple or convenient approach to reliability.

11. Validity data were provided in 65% of the process studies but in only 40% of the outcome studies. The higher proportion of process studies providing validity data (65%) relative to the proportion providing evidence for reliability may not be viewed as a prerequisite to validity by the researchers in this study. Validity data, when obtained in process studies, were collected within the context of the current work and tended to provide evidence for content validity. In the outcome studies, in which validity data were obtained for 40%, more than one approach was employed, including content validity, construct, and criterion related.

Issues and Imperatives in Nursing Process and Outcome Measurement

Results from the analysis of process and outcome work appearing in the 1984 nursing literature are causes of concern. Of most concern is the fact that many of the problems identified by Waltz and Strickland (1981) in an earlier assessment of the state of the art of outcome measurement in nursing were still prevalent, suggesting that little if any improvement has occurred in the measurement principles and practices employed by publishing nurse researchers. More specifically, findings from both studies raise issues regarding the reliability and validity of process and outcome measurement in nursing that must be addressed and resolved if the quality of the nursing process and outcome research is to improve.

As noted, although activities directed toward studying processes and outcomes represent a high proportion of the nursing research published during the period of 1980–1984, activities directed toward measurement of process and outcome variables were quite limited, especially in regard to the measurement of educational variables. It is imperative that nurses give adequate attention to the measurement of both clinical and educational processes and outcomes in order to satisfy internal and external demands for demonstrating the impact of nursing education and practice on health care. Studies on nursing by the Institute of Medicine (1981, 1983) and the National Commission on Nursing (1983) point to the need to adequately assess and measure the educational processes in nursing and their outcomes, so that sound data for national policymaking will be available in nursing education and in the utilization of nursing personnel. The paucity of published research on processes and outcomes in nursing education raises grave concerns regarding the accuracy of available information bases that may be used in such decisions.

It is imperative that two types of reliability and validity be considered in the measurement of process and outcome variables. Foremost, each instrument or method selected or developed for measuring a variable of interest must demonstrate reliability and validity in its own right. Traditionally, reliability and validity efforts, when undertaken, have sought to obtain evidence that a given instrument or method consistently and accurately assigns scores to subjects and that the instrument or method measures what it purports to measure. In 76% of the process studies and 60% of the outcome studies, no reliability data regarding the tools were provided. Equivalently, validity data were supplied in only 65% of the process studies and 40% of the outcome studies.

Each time an instrument or method is employed some error is involved that cannot be eliminated but that can be reduced by using sound approaches to measurement. Measurement error may result from imprecision or systematic bias in the instrument, temporal factors, individual differences at measurement time, or imprecision in the administration or scoring of the measure. Because measurement error may occur as a result of circumstances surrounding the administration of the measure or individual differences at measurement time, reliability and validity investigations conducted on one measurement occasion are not sufficient evidence for reliability and validity when measures are employed on other occasions or with different subjects. Thus, reliability and validity must be determined every time a given measure is employed and moreover with at least two approaches each.

Of equal importance, yet less often considered, is the need to attend to the reliability and validity of the measurement process or approach per se. To increase the probability that the measurement process will yield reliable and valid information, it is necessary (1) to exercise care in the selection of appropriate variables to be measured, (2) whenever possible, to employ multiple instruments or methods to measure any given variable, and (3) to obtain information about any given variable from a number of different sources or perspectives. Pursuing this form of measurement of reliability and validity is largely a function of a well-designed and -executed process.

A major dilemma for nurses regarding the reliability and validity of process and outcome measurement may be the selection of appropriate variables for study. In any given situation, a myriad of variables may be appropriate for process and outcome measurement. That is, in most instances no single concept is likely to represent the outcomes of a particular intervention or process adequately; therefore, the outcomes selected must be based on and be consistent with the conceptual framework that is guiding the research. Unfortunately, findings from this analysis demonstrated that conceptual frameworks were not employed for the tool's development in 100% of the outcome studies and 65% of the process studies. Horn (1980), Atwood (1980), and Blalock (1964) noted that, since process variables by nature are dynamic, a number of concepts may be required for the formulation of a sound definition. These authors also noted that errors usually arise from three sources when a conceptual framework is not formulated to measure process: (1) underspecification or overspecification of key variables, (2) inaccurate or incomplete definitions of key variables, and (3) inaccurate identification of the key variables. Similarly, the study of several key outcome variables and their relationship with each other and the nursing interaction will provide rich information and will more likely further develop the knowledge base regarding the phenomenon of interest than will the study of a single outcome variable.

Another major concern regarding the selection of nursing outcome variables stems from the fact that most outcomes are influenced by many factors beyond these that are the focus of the research. Hence, it is difficult to select outcomes that can be attributed to only one factor. However, in most cases it is possible to select outcomes that can be related temporally to the intervention or process that is the focus of the investigation. Temporally relating variation in outcomes to the expected source of such changes supports the validity and usefulness for the outcome selected. Timing of measurement is therefore important, and outcomes should be selected that are expected to respond to the type of action, interaction, or process that is conducted.

The use of multiple measures of both process and outcome variables can provide more support for reliability and validity in its own right. No single method can be trusted to provide a comprehensive perspective on the phenomenon under study. Since each measure has unique strengths and weaknesses, researchers will benefit if they use a variety of methods and sources, because doing so allows them to capitalize on the strengths of each while also minimizing its weaknesses. Furthermore, when findings are consistent using two or more measures of the same variable(s), evidence for reliability and validity is apparent and the accuracy of decisions made on the basis of results is apt to be high (Waltz, 1984).

In sum, if research investigating the relationship between nursing processes and outcomes is to be based on sound measurement practice, it is imperative that nurses attend to the issues and imperatives related to the selection of appropriate variables for study, the utilization of reliable and valid tools and methods, and the employment of multiple methods to measure a given variable.

Recommendations

Regrettably, considering the results of this assessment of the state of the art of process and outcome measurement in nursing as reflected in the literature in 1984, the same recommendations offered a few years ago remain relevant and thus are reiterated here (Waltz & Strickland, 1981):

1. Nurse researchers should give more attention to the measurement of both clinical and educational processes and outcomes. In addition, the measurement of educational variables needs to be legitimized and stressed as being as important as the measurement of clinical variables.
2. Nurse researchers should broaden their perspective regarding the type of process and outcome measures that are important for study, so that efforts will be more balanced toward the consideration for behavioral and psychological outcomes as well as perceptual and attitudinal phenomena that tend to be too heavily relied upon.
3. Efforts should be made to encourage more use of conceptual frameworks in studies, and consistency between conceptual frameworks and the measures that are employed to operationalize variables.
4. More rigor should be exercised in the application of measurement principles in nursing studies. This goal will more likely be realized if measurement becomes essential content in nursing research courses, as well as a course focus in its own right in nursing graduate programs.
5. Nurses should make a concerted effort to share, modify, and utilize existing tools and measures in a variety of settings and with varied populations. The creation of clearing houses for tools and other measures should facilitate this effort.
6. Nursing research journals should encourage the application of more rigorous measurement principles in articles that are published.
7. More nursing workshops and symposia should be focused on measurement and instrumentation in nursing.

In essence, nurses need to give measurement the attention and support it warrants clinically and educationally if the important goal of documenting the process and outcomes of practice is to be accomplished.

REFERENCES

Atwood, J. R. (1980). A research perspective. *Nursing Research, 29*, 104–108.

Blalock, H. M. (1964). *Causal inferences in nonexperimental research.* Chapel Hill: University of North Carolina Press.

Bloch, D. (1981). Conceptualization of nursing research and nursing sciences. In J. C. McCloskey & H. K. Grace (Eds.), *Current issues in nursing.* Boston: Blackwell.

Bloch, D. (1975). Evaluation of nursing care in terms of process and outcome: Issues in research and quality assurance. *Nursing Research, 24*, 256–263.

Donabedian, A. (1970). Patient care evaluation. *Hospitals, 44*,131–137.

Garfield, E. (1984). Citation patterns in nursing journals, and their most-cited articles. *Current Contents, 27*, 3–12.

Gortner, S. R., Bloch, D., & Phillips, T. P. (1976). Contributions of nursing research to patient care. *Journal of Nursing Administration, 6*(3), 22–28.

Horn, B. J. (1980). Establishing valid and reliable criteria: A researcher's perspective. *Nursing Research, 29*, 88–90.

Institute of Medicine (1981). *Six-month interim report by the committee of the Institute of Medicine for a study of nursing and nursing education.* Washington, DC: National Academy Press.

Institute of Medicine (1983). *Nursing and nursing education: Public policies and private actions.* Washington, DC: National Academy Press.

Martuza, V. R. (1977). *Applying norm-referenced and criterion-referenced measurement in education.* Boston: Allyn & Bacon.

National Commission on Nursing (1983). *Summary report and recommendations.* Chicago: American Hospital Association.

Nunnally, J. C. (1978). *Psychometric Theory.* New York: McGraw-Hill.

Waltz, C. F. (January 1984). *Improving the quality of decisions in nursing education via triangulation.* Paper presented to the Society for Research in Nursing Education, San Francisco.

Waltz, C. F., & Strickland, O. L. (1981). Measurement of nursing outcomes: State-of-the-art as we enter the eighties. In W. E. Field (Ed.), *Measuring outcomes of nursing practice, education, and administration: Proceedings of the First Annual Southern Council on Collegiate Education for Nursing Conference.* Atlanta: Southern Regional Education Board.

Waltz, C. F., Strickland, O. L. & Lenz, E. R. (1984). *Measurement in nursing research.* Philadelphia: Davis.

Comment

Researcher Expertise and Consultation in Instrument Development

SANDRA FERKETICH, Ph.D., R.N.

The preceding chapter features a well-conceived study addressing the issues and imperatives in instrumentation in nursing research. The findings and implications in instrument development were clear, concise, and logically consistent with the orientation and framework posed by the authors. The following comments begin with a brief overview of the study done by Waltz and Strickland, which is followed by a discussion of major concerns that support and complement the study. Special emphasis is placed on fostering researcher expertise and seeking consultation in the process of instrument development.

The study was confined to research on nursing process and outcome management published in three core nursing research journals. The findings can be summarized as indicating that research in nursing process and outcome management was insufficient primarily in three broad categories: (1) area of study, (2) design, and (3) expertise of the researcher. Area of study refers to such findings as a limited number of studies on process and outcome in general and a dearth of studies on education of nurses. Design issues focused on problems such as the lack of a conceptual framework and the lack a of multiple indices of the variables of interest. Lastly, researcher expertise was in question when there was an embarrassing lack of understanding about and attention to the issues of reliability and validity.

The imperatives for nursing, formulated in the preceding chapter, address these three broad categories. To combat the lack of interest in nursing education research, the need to respect educational research is posited. Increased rigor in the education of researchers, the review of work for journal publication, and the expectation of use of a conceptual framework in instrument development are ways to address design problems and lack of researcher expertise. Lastly, the authors called for greater communication of instrumentation results and a greater attention to building on work already available in the field.

In the chapter the lack of attention paid to instrument reliability and validity and the use of researcher-devised instruments for individual studies are cited. The current dilemma in instrumentation concerns the availability and access to adequately tested instruments for a particular construct under study. Researchers are faced with having to use an instrument mismatched with the selected construct or with having to use a new and previously untested but conceptually more sound instrument. Neither solution, of course, is tenable. An instrument that fails to measure the construct helps create a study fraught with validity issues. On the other hand, a researcher who develops an instrument for just one study inadvertently poses many questions regarding measurement error, reliability, and validity.

The issue of expertise of the researcher is pivotal in further explicating the dilemma. The chapter proposes that measurement be a core component in graduate education. Inherent in the decision to include such content is the approval and support of instrument development as the main topic for a dissertation.

It is important that the researcher considering instrument development understand the full extent of efforts that will be necessary. It is worthwhile emphasizing that instrument development is a complex topic. Nunnally (1978) states that adequate measurement starts with careful attention to the identification and definition of the construct. That is, a well-thought-through plan and procedure for construction of the instrument lays the framework for further psychometric work. This, however, is only the foundation, not the entirety of the effort. Further, an instrument should be examined from the perspective of how the instrument behaves internally to itself, considering the preset logic of the construction, and how the instrument behaves in relation to the external world of people and other measures. There are varieties of approaches to reliability and validity, and these may be assessed step by step in separate studies, or a number of approaches may be combined in one study. Whatever the route chosen, however, instrument development requires that many pieces of evidence be amassed.

At this point of considering a plan of action the novice instrument developer is most likely to seek outside assistance. It is, therefore, important to raise the issue of use of consultation related to measurement. There are several facets to this issue: the timing of the consultation, the credentials of the consultant, the preparation of the nurse researcher for the consultation process, and the match between consultant and researcher. It is certainly possible that nurse researchers will reach the point in which consultation on instrument development will be needed in only a minor sense. Currently, for the majority of nurse researchers engaged in instrument development, this is not the case, and quite frequently extensive consultation is necessary.

The timing of the consultation is critical. Suffice it to say that it is not unlike timing for any other research endeavor. Thus, consultation from the very beginning, that is, from the inception of the instrument, is crucial. Manipulation of data with advanced statistical processes to handle lack of power at later points in the instrument development has only the effect of a Band-Aid. The guiding maxim is, "Don't wait or it may be too late."

The credentials of the consultant should be examined. Statisticians, both the true ones and the self-proclaimed, come from varying backgrounds. Most often they diverge widely in basic approaches and areas of application. A consultant with an economics background, for example, may have little expertise in instrument development. While content for analytic procedures can be learned to some extent, a more important and probably more subtle influence is the basic approach to analysis. For the novice instrument developer, selecting a consultant with background preparation in instrumentation is probably more critical than trying to find a variety of sources on new or esoteric approaches.

An additional consideration is the background of the researcher. Statistical analysis is not to be feared, and a basic understanding of analytic procedures is necessary and attainable. It facilitates communication with other scientists, but, more important, it permits researchers to make informed decisions about their work, including decisions about suggestions made by a consultant.

Lastly, the match between consultant and researcher is essential. The consultant needs to provide the expertise the researcher lacks, and the researcher needs to understand where his or her own expertise ends and the need for additional expertise begins. The researcher should know the field of inquiry without equal, and the consultant should have a background broad enough to understand the basic premises of this field of application.

No matter how carefully done or extensive any work is, including instrument development, we must realize that all evidence is still circumstantial. We do not "prove" the efficacy of an instrument, we only support its efficacy in study after study. It behooves the researcher to consider critically the long road to be followed in the careful enumeration and testing of an instrument before starting down the path. If instrument development and its subsequent use in answering a research question are to be worthwhile and contribute to both the developer's work and that of others, then time, patience, and perseverance become essential parts of the program of development. Anything less is an injustice to the researcher and the discipline.

REFERENCES

Nunnally, J. C. (1978). Psychometric theory. *New York: McGraw-Hill.*

16

A Statistician's View on Statistics, Quantitative Methods, and Nursing

DONNA R. BROGAN, Ph.D.

Drawing upon both the literature and my personal experiences as a statistician collaborating with nurse researchers, this chapter presents issues related to (1) common views held by statisticians regarding the use of statistics and quantitative methods in nursing; (2) the teaching of statistics to nursing students; (3) the collaboration between a statistics–biostatistics department and a school of nursing in a university environment; (4) women and quantitative methods; and (5) the regulation of statisticians. It is perhaps informative to describe my background and current involvement in nursing research, as both have been influential in shaping the ideas presented here.

Background and Perspective

I was an undergraduate mathematics major but chose statistics for graduate work because of my interest in applied mathematics. As an undergraduate, I minored in psychology and chemistry, giving me an appreciation of measurement and data collection problems in both the "soft" and "hard" sciences. I have worked primarily in a university setting, both in a school of public health and a school of medicine. My usual activities include teaching graduate statistics courses and collaborative research in medicine, health, and social science.

For 10 years at Emory University I taught research methods and statistics in the master's program at the Nell Hodgson Woodruff School of Nursing. I consulted individually with literally hundreds of graduate nursing students on their master's thesis research and with nursing faculty on research proposals and projects.

My perspectives on the integration of statistics and quantitative methods in nursing are shaped by the following factors: (1) my training in statistics, (2) my teaching and research experience in nursing, (3) my desire for quality teaching of statistics to health professionals, (4) my concern for the appropriate use of statistics in the health sciences, and (5) my commitment to the availability of nondiscriminatory educational and employment opportunities for women.

The Disciplines of Nursing and Statistics

What viewpoint does the statistics discipline have toward the use of statistics in nursing? The response from most statisticians would be the same if any other discipline were substituted for nursing (e.g., engineering, medicine, or political science): Statisticians welcome the use of statistical theory and methods in all disciplines, particularly in a research context.

Nursing has made substantial progress in the research arena since *Nursing Research* appeared in 1952, including more nursing research, more nurses doing research, more clinical or practice-based research, greater theoretical orientation of the research, and more use of sound methodology, including statistics (Brown, Tanner, & Padrick, 1984; Feldman, 1980). Two continuing problems are (1) the lack of a dominant focus on practice-based research and (2) the lack of continued productivity of nurse researchers, who seem to disappear from research into administration (Gortner, 1982; Greenwood, 1984; Moustafa, 1985). Additional problems are (3) the poor quality of statistical analysis and interpretation in the nursing research literature and (4) the assumed "difficulty" in teaching statistics to nursing students (Hinshaw & Schepp, 1984; Johnson, 1984; Ludeman, 1982).

Poor statistical quality in the nursing research literature is addressed in other chapters in this book. It is easy to find examples of misused and abused statistical techniques, as well as misinterpretations of correctly applied statistical techniques in nursing, medical, and health journals (Hooke, 1980). The statistical presentations are not "significantly" better in the higher-prestige journals, such as the *New England Journal of Medicine* and *Nursing Research*. Similar comments hold for the quality of research design and statistical analyses in research proposals. Statistical quality may actually be decreasing over the years as more journals and research funding agencies insist upon statistical analysis and the crucial p-value (Salsburg, 1985) before an article can be published or a research proposal can be funded. In many instances it does not seem to matter if the statistical analysis and the p-value are right or wrong, just that they be present.

The statistics discipline can make important contributions to the research endeavor in nursing, and it is likely that the correct use of statistics, quantitative methods, and research design will further advance nursing's scientific stature. Given that this viewpoint is widely held in nursing, what causes the continued poor quality of statistics in nursing journals and research proposals? Several potential causal factors can be identified, some of which are related to the teaching of statistics to nursing students.

Teaching Statistics to Nursing Students

CONCERNS HELD BY STATISTICIANS

The Subsection on the Teaching of Statistics in the Health Sciences was founded about 15 years ago within the American Statistical Association (ASA) to improve the teaching of statistics to medical students. This group later expanded its interest to nursing and allied health. It has become clear that there is no easy or obvious solution to the problem of teaching introductory statistics to these groups. Medical students usually do not view statistics as useful when they are exposed to it in their undergraduate curriculum, and they rarely study statistics as part of graduate or residency training (Brogan, 1980a). Graduate nursing students, although generally more convinced of the utility of statistics, especially in a research context, often are afraid of mathematical sciences and typically are quantitatively weak (Bindler & Bayne, 1984; Johnson, 1984; Ludeman, 1982; Muhlenkamp, 1981). Graduate students in the allied health professions are similar to nurses in terms of math anxiety and quantitative ability.

Thus, statisticians have a continuing concern, but no definitive answers, regarding the teaching of introductory statistics to graduate nursing students. The issue itself is complex and there are various aspects to it. Those aspects are now reviewed. It should be emphasized that the comments to follow are focused primarily on the introductory statistics courses, often at the master's level, rather than on the advanced statistics courses that may be included in doctoral nursing programs.

COURSE CONTENT AND CONTEXT

The approach to teaching introductory statistics needs to be tailored to the particular student group. First, the mathematical level at which the course is taught needs to be consistent with the students' background. Nursing students typically are less skilled quantitatively than engineering students, with nurses rarely having a calculus background and engineers typically being prepared in advanced calculus. Second, the course content and context should reflect the research work setting in which statistics is likely to be used by the students in their future careers. The content–context may vary substantially over student groups, since different types of statistical techniques are commonly used in each discipline.

The introductory course should use nursing examples, preferably from the nursing research literature. If time permits, students should receive guided practice in reading journal articles, particularly the research design and statistical aspects. Although some statisticians would argue that introductory statistics can be taught independently of subject matter and discipline, with diverse examples from accounting to zoology, this approach does not work well with quantitatively weak students. It seems overwhelming to these students to cope with the mathematical–algebraic issues in the statistics course in addition to new concepts and terminology from other disciplines. Firmly grounding the introductory statistics course in nursing examples and selecting the content to be reflective of techniques commonly used in nursing helps combat some of the mathematical–statistics anxiety and negative attitude that usually are present among nursing students (Ludeman, 1981).

Introductory statistics is best taught to graduate students in conjunction with research methods. This approach makes it easier for students to see the utility of statistics (Brogan & Kutner, 1986), since they will do research for their graduate degree and may be research investigators or consumers in their future careers. This link between statistics and research is harder to establish on the undergraduate level than on the graduate level because undergraduates have less firm choices of academic majors and their programs place less or no emphasis on research.

The statistics course and the research methods course can be taught in both orders. To teach research methods first, followed by statistics, is perhaps preferable because the statistical technique can be presented as appropriate analyses for one or more of the research designs previously studied. However, the research methods–statistics sequence advocated here may also pose problems. For instance, a typical objective of a methods course is to be able to read and critique the research literature. It is difficult to understand journal articles when one has little or no skill at reading tables or graphics and no understanding of basic statistical terminology. A proved solution is to teach these basic statistical concepts in the research methods course. However, one should also consider blending research methods and statistics into a two-quarter or one-semester introductory course. Detailed recommendations on course objectives and content for introductory research methods and statistics in nursing are given in Brogan (1980b) with student course evaluations reported in Brogan (1980a).

COURSE LIMITATIONS

An important aspect of the introductory statistics course is realization of its limitations by both the nursing students and the nursing faculty. It is without question impossible to give graduate students a thorough training in statistics in a one-semester course (Brogan & Kutner, 1986). One-semester introductory statistics courses that claim to enable students to undertake statistical analyses independently are misleading to students. Such students are likely to use over and over again the few statistical techniques they learned, whether or not they are appropriate for the situation at hand.

A two-semester introductory statistics sequence offers greater opportunities. Within the context of such a sequence, it is reasonable to teach several statistical techniques that students can do independently. More important, such a sequence offers time to teach students how to recognize the situations that warrant statistical consultation. Thus, a one-semester introductory statistics course needs to include a strong message always to consult a competent statistician on research design and statistical analysis plans. After a two-semester introductory statistics sequence, students may be better able to judge in what instances statistical consultation is needed and what problems they should be able to tackle confidently themselves (Brogan & Kutner, 1986).

QUANTITATIVE ABILITY OF STUDENTS

A major aspect of teaching introductory statistics to graduate nursing students is the low level of quantitative background and ability, often accompanied by mathematics–statistics anxiety (Bindler & Bayne, 1984; Johnson, 1984; Ludeman, 1982; Muhlenkamp, 1981). It is difficult to teach the foundations of statistics accurately to someone who has difficulty with signed numbers and high school algebra. Such students may be able to memorize enough to pass an introductory statistics course, and they may even be able to run an analysis of variance in SPSS, but it is unlikely they will understand what they are doing. It does more harm than good to the disciplines of both nursing and statistics to teach students this way.

But why are nursing students, and others as well, often educated so that they can do calculations or run statistical software packages but are unable to use and interpret statistical analyses correctly? Is it because they are weak quantitatively? That is only part of the problem, much of which can be overcome by requiring appropriate math prerequisites and then teaching in a manner that minimizes math anxiety. Alternatively, the minimum mathematical skills, basically college algebra, can be incorporated into the introductory statistics course. This latter approach, however, requires more time for the introductory statistics course or less coverage of statistical topics.

BEHAVIOR PATTERNS OF STUDENTS

Although weak quantitative skills is a major factor in "mislearning" statistics, there are additional factors that may be unique to nursing. One factor is nurses' apparent discomfort with the entire notion of uncertainty. As noted also by Wilson (1982), nursing students seem upset by the idea that inferential statistics will not always give the correct answer, that is, the right answer. Those who really understand the concepts of Type I Error and confidence interval are unsettled and unnerved by them, perhaps because these concepts run counter to their previous training. Further, nursing students seem to want definite rules for choosing a research design, for analyzing data, and for drawing conclusions. This "certainty" behavior may be desirable or necessary in clinical environments, but research and the use of statistics are more creative processes where it is difficult to make always or never statements.

Related to the apparent desire for certainty is the reaction to authority. Graduate nursing students seem distressed when it is stated that some of the published nursing, medical, and health research is useless—and perhaps dangerous—because it is so poorly done (Hinshaw & Schepp, 1984). It is hard to dispel notions like "if it's published, it must be correct and true," or, "it must be accurate if it's on a computer printout." Nursing is changing in this area (MacPherson, 1983), but there still is some distance to go.

It warrants asking to what extent these behavior patterns are associated with or perhaps caused by (1) selective entry into nursing, (2) socialization into the nursing profession, and/or (3) socialization into the female role by society (Young, 1984), particularly the school system (Kutner & Brogan, 1976). However, various authors mention these behaviors in the continuing concern for more productivity among nurse researchers (e.g., Downs, 1985; Lia-Hoagberg, 1985; Roncoli, 1985).

COURSE INSTRUCTOR

One of the most important issues in teaching introductory statistics to nursing students is *who* teaches the course. In some instances the introductory course is taught by a statistician, defined as a person whose primary discipline is statistics. Perhaps more frequently the course is taught by instructors from other disciplines, such as nursing, psychology, sociology, or education. These instructors typically studied statistics, some of them having a minor or second major in statistics at the graduate level. Unfortunately, some of these instructors are not well trained in statistics and do not have an adequate understanding of its basic theoretical and conceptual foundations. Their own misconceptions and misinterpretations are transmitted to students, who often end up more misinformed than the instructor. Frequently this is repeated in an incestuous fashion as graduate students taught by these instructors enter academia in their own discipline and teach what they believe to be statistics to the following generation of graduate students.

Because of this scenario, perhaps more common in other disciplines than in nursing, applied statistics courses, particularly introductory courses, are best taught by persons who have applied and theoretical graduate training in statistics. These persons usually have statistics as a primary graduate discipline. However, not all statisticians would be good teachers of introductory statistics, particularly with quantitatively weak audiences. A mathematical statistician may not be a good choice to teach an introductory course because this instructor and the graduate nursing students rarely look at the topic from the same perspective.

In addition to recommending that statistics instructors have adequate theoretical and applied training, it is also desirable that instructors for introductory courses be active as applied statisticians, using statistics to plan and implement research projects and to manage, analyze, and interpret data. Several statisticians work in both the applied and theoretical modes, using their applied experience to suggest problems for further theoretical research.

Given the recommendation that an applied statistician teach an introductory statistics course to nurses, it is necessary that the statistician be knowledgeable about nursing research. The statistician should be interested in nursing and committed to make any extra effort needed to present the course in a nursing context. Unfortunately, not all statisticians are willing to do so. In some statistics departments the reward system is geared not to teaching nonstatistics majors, but to teaching advanced statistics courses for statistics majors and publishing statistical research. Thus, a statistician who "goes the extra mile" for the nursing students may suffer opportunity cost (e.g., one less statistical publication that year).

INTERMEDIATE AND ADVANCED STATISTICS COURSES

The preceding discussion and recommendations are specific to an introductory statistics course at the master's level in nursing. Although I have no personal experience in teaching intermediate and advanced statistics courses to doctoral students in nursing, I will modify my preceding recommendations for this situation based on my teaching experience in disciplines other than nursing. First, these statistics courses should be taught by a statistician with both applied and theoretical training in statistics. Second, it is not necessary that the courses be primarily oriented toward nursing. After one or two introductory statistics courses, nursing students should understand the foundations and basic concepts of statistics and be able to apply to nursing the statistical techniques learned in other contexts, such as social science or biology. Third, math anxiety and poor quantitative skills should be less of a problem at this level, since the doctoral nursing students should have adequate quantitative skills to begin with or should take the necessary mathematics courses so as to satisfy the prerequisites for intermediate and advanced statistics.

A common theme in this book is the recommendation that doctoral-level nurses be knowledgeable in statistical areas, such as time series, multivariate analysis, log-linear models, and path analysis or causal modeling. Although this would certainly be desirable, it may prove unrealistic for most nurses, because few statisticians are knowledgeable in all these areas. Statistics is similar to other disciplines in that it has specialty areas, and doctoral-level statisticians tend to specialize in one or two areas because it is impossible to keep current in several statistical specialties. It is important for doctoral nurses to be aware of the various statistical specialties and the focus of each one, perhaps learning a few commonly used techniques in each specialty. This will allow doctoral nurses to identify what statistical specialty, if any, is likely to be useful in a given situation and thus to make the search for an appropriate statistical consultant more fruitful.

Collaboration Between a Statistics Department and a School of Nursing

INTRODUCTORY STATISTICS COURSE

The preceding comments lead naturally into how a school of nursing and a statistics or biostatistics department can cooperate toward the objective of graduate nursing students learning and applying introductory, intermediate, and advanced statistics. Unless the school of nursing has a qualified faculty member trained in theoretical and applied statistics, it most likely will seek out someone in the statistics–biostatistics department to teach. Note that it usually is not productive for a school of nursing to seek a statistics instructor from such departments as sociology, education, or psychology, since these faculty members typically are not trained in the theory of statistics.

The school of nursing needs to make clear to the statistics–biostatistics department that it wants an applied introductory statistics course with nursing orientation and nursing examples. If the nursing student body is large enough to form a complete class or section, then the school might be successful in getting the statistics–biostatistics department to orient an entire section or course specifically to nursing. If there are not enough students for this approach, then the nursing students can be combined with students in similar disciplines, so that quantitative skills will be homogeneous and course examples will be relevant to most students. It is feasible to combine students in nursing, physical therapy, occupational therapy, community health, and health education. In addition to overlapping subject matters, these groups have similar quantitative skills.

If the school of nursing is working with a statistics instructor who has not taught nursing students before, it is important to alert the instructor to the nursing research journals, identify the most common research methodologies used in nursing, and suggest that some nonparametric techniques be covered, since many of the measurement scales used in nursing are ordinal.

If a school of nursing wants an introductory statistics course blended with or in combination with research methods, few existing courses may be offered in statistics–biostatistics departments that meet these objectives. Many statistics departments have not emphasized research design and the scientific method in their introductory statistics courses, although this is changing currently. Thus, if a school of nursing wishes an introductory sequence that blends research methods and statistics, it may need to negotiate a special arrangement with the statistics–biostatistics department. The latter may or may not be interested in working with the former; it depends on their orientation and the local system of academic rewards and funding.

INTERMEDIATE AND ADVANCED STATISTICS COURSES

Not all schools of nursing have the resources to offer intermediate and advanced applied statistics courses. Hence, they might have to rely on regular course offerings of the statistics–biostatistics departments on campus. At this level it is not crucial that the statistics courses be specifically oriented to nursing. With a good introductory sequence, the nursing students should understand the basic concepts of statistics and how they are relevant to nursing. Further, those nursing students pursuing intermediate or advanced statistics courses presumably would have the necessary quantitative skills required as prerequisites for these courses.

Women and Quantitative Methods

Educators in the United States are concerned about the low level of mathematical and quantitative ability at all stages of education and in the larger society among both men and women. However, women choose a career in mathematics, statistics, and computer science at a rate much less than that of men (Kutner & Brogan, 1985), a major reason being that girls choose fewer math courses than boys in high school and college. Further, math anxiety is more prevalent among girls and women than among boys and men. It also has been documented over many generations that elementary school girls perform as well as or better than elementary school boys in virtually all subjects, but in junior high school and high school boys begin consistently to outperform girls in mathematics and science (Fishbein, 1982; Kutner & Brogan, 1985).

Since nursing science is a discipline wherein many of its members are female, the issue of women and quantitative methods is relevant. The long-term solution to this problem may be a long time coming. In the meantime those who teach required quantitative methods courses to nurses need to take this phenomenon into account. When teaching introductory statistics to master's level nursing students it is important to deal with the math anxiety that is known to be there. It helps to explain what all statistical symbols mean and to emphasize that statisticians use symbols as a short-hand to avoid writing a lot of words. It also is helpful to explain most algebraic steps and to teach students to state in English what each symbolic expression says. This approach, however, is too elementary for the few students in the class who have had calculus, and they are likely to find this approach irritating. One proposed solution is to recommend that the quantitatively skilled students take an introductory statistics course outside the school of nursing.

Many women have math anxiety. This phenomenon occurs to a large enough extent in nursing that it needs to be recognized and incorporated into any teaching of quantitative methods to this group, particularly in an introductory course. This is not to say that courses for nurses should be watered down; that approach recognizes the math anxiety and weak quantitative background but does nothing about it. Furthermore, such "cookbook" courses are at high risk of teaching misconceptions about statistics. It is important to face and reduce the math anxiety and quantitative weakness, through either including algebra as a component of introductory statistics or requiring appropriate prerequisites.

Note that this section of the chapter is based on the implied assumption that it is desirable and/or scientific to be quantitatively skilled and oriented. Thus, the issue becomes how to get the nursing discipline up to this standard, which undoubtedly is underwritten in one form or another by most statisticians and quantitative scientists. However, some of the nursing literature states that this goal, although laudable, may be counter-productive if pursued without question. Several nurse researchers argue for going beyond the quantitative method, or at least supplementing it with a more qualitative approach (MacPherson, 1983; Omery, 1983; Swanson & Chenitz, 1982; Tinkle & Beaton, 1983). It is important to be aware of this viewpoint in nursing and other scientific disciplines as well.

Regulation of Statisticians

The widespread availability of inexpensive statistical software packages to run on inexpensive microcomputers will increase the misuse and abuse of statistics dramatically, not only in nursing but in all disciplines.

This will occur because more people will be able to do their own statistical analyses rather than going to someone else. Many of these people will not be trained in the correct use of statistics. They will respond to software advertisements that say, "You don't need to know anything about statistics or computing to run this statistical software package." That ad probably is true. However, the ad *does not* state that one needs to know something about research design and statistics to choose the appropriate statistical technique for the given situation. Then one needs to know something about statistics to interpret the calculations that the program produces on the computer screen or computer printout. Finally, one needs to know something about statistics to know if the output makes sense or whether it is garbage, because some error was made in the data input, in the commands input, or in the statistical software itself (Hinshaw & Schepp, 1984).

Personally, I am being led to strongly consider the proposal that statisticians be licensed, certified, or regulated in some manner. Although I understand that regulation of any sort presents many issues and potential problems, it is also my concern as a statistician to reduce the frequent misuses and misinterpretations of statistical techniques. Regulation is not a popular position within the American Statistical Association (ASA). Concern for the ethical practice of statistics first appeared in the 1940s in the United States with rekindled interest in the 1970s and 1980s (Ellenberg, 1983; Gibbons, 1973), culminating in the recent ASA draft publication of "Ethical Guidelines for Statistical Practice" (1983). There is a difference of opinion within the ASA whether ethical guidelines are even needed (Schneiderman, 1984). Among those who generally support a code of ethics, there is controversy over whether certification is needed to make the code workable (Greenhouse, 1983; Roberts, 1983). Nonetheless, a small group has argued for certification before and after the recently ASA published ethical guidelines (Boen & Smith, 1985). Although to date the regulation–certification issue has not been addressed seriously by the ASA, it is a topic whose time has come for consideration and debate.

References

Bindler, R., & Bayne, T. (1984). Do baccalaureate students possess basic mathematics proficiency? *Journal of Nursing Education, 23*, 192–197.

Boen, J. & Smith, H. (1985). Should statisticians be certified? *The American Statistician, 39*, 113–114.

Brogan, D. R. (1980a). A program of teaching and consultation in research methods and statistics for graduate students in nursing. *The American Statistician, 34*, 26–33.

Brogan, D. R. (1980b). An integrated approach to training in research methodology and statistics. *International Journal of Nursing Studies, 17*, 101–106.

Brogan, D. R., & Kutner, M. (1986). Graduate service statistics courses: What, to whom, and by whom? In *Proceedings of the American Statistical Association: Statistical Education*. Washington, DC: The Association.

Brown, S., Tanner, A., & Padrick, P. (1984). Nursing's search for scientific knowledge. *Nursing Research, 33*, 26–32.

Downs, S. (1985). Is there life after the doctorate? *Nursing Research, 34*, 133.

Ellenberg, H. (1983). Ethical guidelines for statistical practice: A historical perspective. *The American Statistician, 37*, 1–4.

Ethical guidelines for statistical practice: Report of the Ad Hoc Committee on Professional Ethics (1983). *The American Statistician, 37*, 5–20.

Feldman, H. R. (1980). Nursing research in the 1980's: Issues and implications. *Advances in Nursing Science, 3*(1), 85–92.

Fishbein, E. G. (1982). Female gender as a variable in the educational process: A review. *Journal of Nursing Education, 21*(5), 43–48.

Gibbons, J. D. (1973). A question of ethics. *The American Statistician, 27*, 72–76.

Gortner, S. R. (1982). Researchmanship: Structures for research productivity. *Western Journal of Nursing Research, 4*, 119–123.

Greenhouse, S. W. (1983). Comment on "Ethical Guidelines for Statistical Practice: Report of the Ad Hoc Committee on Professional Ethics." *The American Statistician, 37*, 15–16.

Greenwood, J. (1984). Nursing research: A position paper. *Journal of Advanced Nursing, 9*, 77-82.

Hinshaw, A. S., & Schepp, K. (1984). How to recognize garbage when you see it. *Western Journal of Nursing Research, 6*, 126–130.

Hooke, R. (1980). Getting people to use statistics properly. *The American Statistician, 34*, 39–42.

Johnson, J. M. (1984). Strategies for teaching nursing research: Strategies for including statistical concepts in a course in research methodology for baccalaureate nursing students. *Western Journal of Nursing Research, 6*, 259–264.

Kutner, N. G., & Brogan, D. R. (April, 1985). *A comparative examination of women in selected quantitative fields*. Paper presented at the Annual Meeting of the Southern Sociological Society, Charlotte, NC.

Kutner, N. G., & Brogan, D. R. (1976). Sources of sex discrimination in educational systems: A conceptual model. *Psychology of Women Quarterly, 1*, 50–69.

Lia-Hoagberg, B. (1985). Comparison of professional activities of nurse doctorates and other women academics. *Nursing Research, 34*, 155–159.

Ludeman, R. (1981). First class sessions are crucial to success. *Western Journal of Nursing Research, 3*, 116–117.

Ludeman, R. (1982). Experimental learning in data analysis. *Western Journal of Nursing Research, 4*, 124–126.

MacPherson, K. I. (1983). Feminist methods: A new paradigm of nursing research. *Advances in Nursing Science, 5*(2), 17–25.

Moustafa, N. G. (1985). Nursing research from 1977 to 1981. *Western Journal of Nursing Research, 7*, 349–356.

Muhlenkamp, A. F. (1981). Densensitization of the research phobia: Instructor as therapist. *Western Journal of Nursing Research, 3*, 305–309.

Omery, A. (1983). Phenomenology: A method for nursing research. *Advances in Nursing Science, 5*(2), 49–63.

Roberts, H. V. (1983). Comment on "Ethical Guidelines for Statistical Practice: Report of the Ad Hoc Committee on Professional Ethics." *The American Statistician, 37*, 18.

Roncoli, M. (1985). Letter to the editor. *Nursing Research, 34*, 65.

Salsburg, D. S. (1985). The religion of statistics as practiced in medical journals. *The American Statistician, 39*, 220–223.

Schneiderman, M. A. (1984). Letter to the editor: Code of ethics. *The American Statistician, 38*, 160.

Swanson, J. M., & Chenitz, C. W. (1982). Why qualitative research in nursing? *Nursing Outlook, 30*, 241–245.

Tinkle, M. B., & Beaton, J. L. (1983). Toward a new view of science: Implications for nursing research. *Advances in Nursing Science. 5*(2), 27–36.

Wilson, H. S. (1982). Teaching research in nursing: Issues and strategies. *Western Journal of Nursing Research, 4*, 365–377.

Young, K. J. (1984). Professional commitment of women in nursing. *Western Journal of Nursing Research, 6*, 11–26.

Acknowledgments

Preparation of this paper was partially supported by grant RII-8503517 from the Visiting Professorship for Women Program of National Science Foundation and by the Biostatistics Department at The University of Michigan.

Comment

Adding to the Statistician's Views and Concerns

BALDEO K. TANEJA, Ph.D.

Scientific research is a process of guided investigation and learning. The object of statistics is to make that process as efficient as possible. Statistical techniques, if not applied to the real-world problems for their understanding, will lose their importance and appear to be mere deductive exercises. But these techniques must be used with great care if they are to achieve any reliable and meaningful results. Most valuable aspects of statistical techniques are underlying assumptions and experimental designs. Any violation of assumptions should be checked, and their practical consequences should be studied carefully. Conclusions can be drawn easily from a well-designed experiment using elementary techniques, but even the most sophisticated statistical analysis cannot salvage an ill-designed experiment. So the researcher should be reasonably sure about the validity of underlying assumptions and the appropriateness of the design when using statistical techniques.

The abundance of abuse and misuse of statistics that we see in the research literature is there because of either a mismatch between a design and the technique or a violation of the assumptions behind the technique being used. Keeping these things in mind would minimize such malpractice of statistics in research, not only in the field of nursing, but in other areas of scientific investigation as well. Correct use of statistics will greatly improve the professional character of nursing, or of any other discipline.

The preceding chapter accurately illuminates the reasons for the continuing poor showing of statistics in nursing research. Cited were (1) low level of mathematical–quantitative ability of nursing students, (2) lack of understanding of statistical concepts and principles, (3) lack of realization of the limitations of statistics, (4) inadequate contents of statistics courses, and (5) poor teaching of statistics courses.

One reason should be added. It relates to the collaboration between the statistician and the nurse researcher. A successful working relationship requires that both of them listen to each other and reach complete agreement on the project. To solve a problem, one has to understand it and define it first. That usually means listening to each other carefully, which is something that many have never learned to do. All real problems have idiosyncrasies that must be appreciated before statistical methods of tackling them can be adopted. Being too hasty can result in mistakes, such as obtaining the right answer to the wrong problem ("an error of the third kind?").

Nurses taking statistics tend to be hardworking, but also intimidated by quantitative analysis, because they do not have enough training in mathematics. This lack of mathematical–quantitative ability makes it difficult for them to understand the concepts and principles behind statistical techniques. Yet it *is* possible to understand statistical concepts and principles without having mathematical sophistication. Even more important than learning about statistical techniques is the development of what might be called a capability of thinking statistically, and realization of the limitations of statistics. It takes a great deal of effort on the part of an instructor to convey these facets of statistics while bypassing most mathematical details, especially while also staying in the race of "doing research and publishing papers." It is indeed a very challenging job.

Teaching statistics to nurses is very different from teaching statistics to engineering students, simply because of different mathematical background and research application situations. Although a particular technique, concept, or principle can be explained concisely to the engineering students with the help of mathematical symbols and formulas, the same material has to be explained to the nurses using other means, such as graphs, pictures, models, detailed word descriptions, and so on.

The following three-step course sequence for teaching statistics to nurses might perhaps maximize their learning and subsequent application:

a. The first step is to introduce elementary statistics to the students, using lots of examples from nursing. This introductory course may include descriptive statistics, parametric and nonparametric testing of hypotheses in one- and two-sample situations, correlation, and regression.

b. The second step would involve discussing research methods and designs. This may include definition of the problem along with variables and hypotheses, questionnaire designs and interviewing techniques, selection of appropriate designs, reliability and validity of instruments, interpreting and communicating the results.

c. The third step is to show more involved methodologies to students, including advanced experimental designs and multivariate techniques. They should be trained in using statistical packages correctly at this stage.

At each step, published articles from nursing research journals should be discussed in class.

Most nursing students would get a pretty good idea of applications and limitations of statistical techniques to nursing research after undergoing the preceding course work. However, they will not become statisticians. So it would be to their benefit to consult a statistician when they are involved in serious research projects that need some statistical analysis; regrettably, sometimes they do not. Consultation would ensure proper use of statistics in their research, as well as make them comfortable in discussing their research issues with statisticians. This intellectual contact would stimulate both the researcher and the statistician. Of course, ideally, a statistician should be involved in the project from the very beginning.

The recommendation that statisticians be licensed, certified, or regulated in some manner is well taken. Personally, I have seen much statistical malpractice in published research, industry, and law cases. I have personally met with people who call themselves "statisticians" but who do not know what statistics really is. To screen these individuals out of the statistics profession, there has to be some sort of licensing or certification of statisticians.

PART 4

Conclusion and Summary

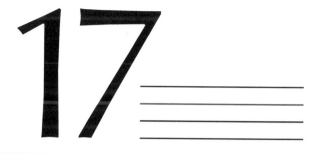

Statistics and Quantitative Methods in Nursing Summarized: Issues and Strategies for the Future

JOYCE J. FITZPATRICK, Ph.D., F.A.A.N.
IVO L. ABRAHAM, Ph.D., R.N.
DEBORAH M. NADZAM, Ph.D., R.N.

This chapter presents a global summary of issues identified in the previous chapters and comments. This summary will serve as the basis for making specific recommendations for the future, both immediate and long range. The issues identified and the recommendations made should be seen as the basis for further discussion. The intent of this chapter is to intensify the considerations about statistics and quantitative methods within the discipline of nursing presented throughout this book.

Issues Within Nursing

Four key issues can be identified; they include (1) delineation of the content of the discipline; (2) delineation of modes of inquiry for the discipline; (3) nature of the educational process, including content and process of socialization; and (4) research collaboration within the discipline.

DELINEATION OF CONTENT OF THE DISCIPLINE

There is consensus within the discipline that the paradigm focus is on the health dimensions of person-environment interaction. Further, there is agreement that nurses, as professionals, intervene with persons in relation to their health. Although, in fact, agreement on the basic discipline concepts of person, environment, health, and nursing has evolved, we have not reached a consensus at the next stage of conceptualization. Thus, there is great diversity in how these basic concepts are defined. Consequently, the varied definitions lead to diverse relational statements. Such diversity is reflected in the apparent disparity across conceptual models. Less frequently, the argument has been advanced that there are more similarities than differences across conceptualizations. The educational model mandates scientific content that is discipline-specific. Although we may choose to continue the debate regarding the basic and/or applied nature of nursing science for academic purposes, it also is imperative that we place high priority on the delineation of the content of the discipline.

DELINEATION OF MODES OF INQUIRY FOR THE DISCIPLINE

Much debate currently exists within the discipline regarding the modes of inquiry most salient to achieving the goals of the discipline. There seems to be no logical argument against multiple modes of inquiry. The decision points occur in areas of emphasis and priority in relation to long- and short-range goals. It is critical that we establish credibility as nurse scientists. Given this short-term, high-priority goal, we would choose to focus on modes of inquiry that not only answer our research questions, but also are widely accepted within the scientific community at large (Fitzpatrick & Abraham, 1987). At the same time we must maintain a scientific position of searching for new and ever deeper problems for investigation. Our research and our methods must be as rigorous as possible in relation to all modes of inquiry, for such scientific rigor and credibility will buy freedom for more diverse methods of inquiry.

NATURE OF THE EDUCATIONAL PROCESS

Quality in the research content of graduate programs, especially the Ph.D. in nursing programs, is essential. Various methods should be used to achieve such quality, including, for example, pre- and postdoctoral fellowships, required research assistantships, and joint faculty–student research projects. Models that have been successful in the more established scientific disciplines should be put in place immediately. The faculty reward systems in university schools of nursing should be directly focused on research and scholarly productivity. Further, we must question our own professional ethics in permitting the proliferation of Ph.D. programs in schools without strong researchers or research goals. Review and accreditation by a professional group would seem warranted. Beyond the issue of educational content is the concern about socialization (Fitzpatrick & Abraham, 1987). We must move quickly to educate professionals into the true professional role and scientists into the true scientist role. Such an endeavor will require concerted effort to change our educational programs at all levels.

RESEARCH COLLABORATION

Many models of research collaboration can be encouraged. Both collaboration within the discipline and across disciplinary boundaries should be promoted. To be successful in any level of collaboration, however, one must be confident of one's own knowledge and credentials.

Strategies for the Future

In response to these and other issues central to the integration of statistics and quantitative methods in nursing, we are prepared to make the following summary recommendations:

1. The development of a *spirit of research* in academic centers should be fostered. It is important for those who have made careers of research to communicate to colleagues and students that research is fun.
2. All scientists should be encouraged to mount *programs of research.* The research developments sparked by such initiatives as the Nursing Research Emphasis Grant for Doctoral Programs in Nursing by the USPHS Division of Nursing should be continued in a systematic manner and should be complemented by similar initiatives.
3. Researchers must be *prepared rigorously.* The limited resource of nurse scientists and well-prepared faculty should be pooled, and the focus should be on the further development of the outstanding research programs. Not only must the future generation of nurse scientists be well prepared in advanced quantitative methods and statistics, but they must also be knowledgeable about the basic disciplinary content. Nurse researchers must have a firm grasp of the theoretical and clinical nursing dimensions of the discipline to advance our knowledge base.
4. We must explore *new methods of measurement* of the phenomena for study. Instrument development should be included as necessary content in doctoral programs in nursing.
5. Bridges toward *content integration* should be developed. This includes development of bridges between theory and research, qualitative and quantitative research, and statistics and clinical nursing. Further, content development should be focused on both theory-generating approaches to science and the research models that are directly relevant to nursing practice.
6. Every effort should be initiated to *socialize future scientists* into the research mode.
7. Efforts to *critique the research* that has already been completed should be encouraged. *The Annual Review of Nursing Research* series has served as an important vehicle for such scholarly integrated reviews.
8. Nurse researchers must become the *image* builders for nursing research, representing their work to the public and scientific communities. There are multiple forums to publicly declare the goals and activities of nurse researchers. Also, students must be oriented to this aspect of their careers.

9. Administrative structures should be designed to reward scholarship. Research productivity must be encouraged and rewarded, and positive pressures exerted by a community of scholars. Research activity must be viewed as an integral part of the role of faculty members and must be integrated into practice settings.

REFERENCES

Fitzpatrick, J. J., & Abraham, I. L. (1987). Towards the socialization of scholars and scientists. *Nurse Educator*, *12*(3), 23–35.

Comment

Fostering "The Burning Yearning for Learning"

HARRIET H. WERLEY, Ph.D., F.A.A.N.

The summary statement on statistics and quantitative methods in nursing in this final chapter is helpful in its enumeration and discussion of four key issues identified from the different chapters. Presented here are selective comments on portions of the recommendations made in the chapter.

Regarding the issue of delineation of modes of inquiry, it is indeed critical for nurses to establish their credibility as nurse scientists, not only within nursing but also within the scientific community at large. It is this scientific community that will judge nurse scientists, serve as peer reviewers on research proposals submitted for funding, review credentials for promotion and tenure, and generally judge the product of nurses' scientific endeavors—that is, the caliber of the research conducted and publication of the findings. Nurses' research methods must be acceptable to the scientific community generally, for "good" science is the same regardless of the discipline involved.

The statement that accreditation of Ph.D. nursing programs would seem warranted merits emphasis. Through the years this has been avoided; one wonders why, when other disciplines do not seem to have any problems with their employing accreditation as a quality control measure. For example, in psychology, the American Psychological Association (APA) accredits its clinical psychology, counseling, and school psychology Ph.D. programs, or combinations of these. The APA does not, however, accredit its scientists' programs. Accreditation of nursing Ph.D. programs might help to stop the proliferation of Ph.D. programs in schools of nursing with an inadequate number of research-productive faculty with funded research programs who can serve as mentors for students. Students are shortchanged when new Ph.D. programs are established in schools of nursing that do not have appropriate numbers of research-qualified and research-productive faculty who can serve as both research and nursing content mentors, because of their extensive research experience.

As to the collaboration issue, within nursing collaboration seems to be taking place on a wider scale than previously. However, collaboration across disciplines is not found as frequently as one might anticipate. One must be confident in one's own knowledge and credentials for successful participation in collaborative efforts to ensue. With faculty developing further as research-productive scientists, no doubt there will be an increase in across-discipline collaboration.

Regarding the recommendation to foster a *spirit of research* in academic centers, it is important that nurses communicate that research is fun and exciting. I am reminded here of something Bernard G. Greenberg (1962, p. 4) shared with us many years ago at a two-week nursing research conference, conducted at the Walter Reed Army Institute of Research (WRAIR) early in 1959. In discussing the definition of research and the differentiation between the education and research processes, he told us there was an added ingredient essential to the research process and that was "the burning yearning for learning" and not "the burning yearning for earning." It is that accretion of answers to research questions that helps to develop the science of nursing.

In a similar vein, regarding the recommendation to encourage nurse scientists to develop programs of research, I am reminded of something Margaret Arnstein (1962) said at the same WRAIR Nursing Research Conference. She spoke of nurses' early research efforts as something like dropping cookies on a cookie sheet—there was no connection between them. In a nursing research program effort, one project would be built upon the other and the expansion of knowledge would be more cohesive.

To implement the recommendation regarding new methods of measurement and the development and refinement of quantitative methods specific to nursing research, we may need to reexamine some prerequisites for research preparation, having to do with mathematics and computer science, so that students can understand and handle measurement principles and quantitative methods.

The recommendation that graduate students learn the research ropes through assistantships reminds me of an article in *Science* in which White (1970) described how a mentor and protégé work together. She enumerated the many things the protégé learns from the mentor in the process of working together on the professor's research program. She said it was the kind of learning that was "caught" not "taught"; that is, one learns the research ropes by being involved in the research of one's mentor.

Regarding recommendation involving the *Annual Review of Nursing Research* and its scholarly reviews, we (the editors) have stressed that authors are not simply to catalogue research that was done, but to critique it. All authors are furnished with a copy of Cooper's (1982) article on critical, integrative reviews, and we have been told by the authors that it was helpful. Cooper has expanded his writing in this area, as evidenced by the fact that more recently he has had a book published on the topic of critical review (Cooper, 1984).

The recommendation related to administrative structures, research productivity, and viewing research as an integral part of faculty role is well taken. Nurses are getting better about not talking so much about research in terms of release time. Research should be viewed as a proportionate time of faculty functioning, and one's role activities should be planned accordingly. Professors do not speak of release time for teaching, so why speak of release time for research, if both are aspects of proper faculty functioning? However, it is well known that when the pressures of workload increase, it usually is the research that is crowded out of faculty functioning. One can question, however, whether that may not also reflect the faculty members' commitment to research. There must be time for thinking, discussion, study, and so on, if one is to maintain progress in one's research program and at the same time keep abreast of developments in statistics and quantitative methods essential to one's research, to say nothing of also keeping abreast of the content area being evolved through the research findings that contribute to nursing's expanding knowledge base.

REFERENCES

Arnstein, M. G. (1962). Research in public health nursing. In H. H. Werley (Ed.), *Report on nursing research conference, 24 February–7 March 1959* (held at Walter Reed Army Institute of Research). Washington, DC: U.S. Government Printing Office.

Cooper, H. M. (1982). Scientific guidelines for conducting integrative research reviews. *Review of Educational Research, 52,* 291–302.

Cooper, H. M. (1984). *The integrative research review: A systematic approach.* Beverly Hills, CA: Sage.

Greenberg, B. G. (1962). The philosophy and methods of research. In H. H. Werley (Ed.), *Report on nursing research conference, 24 February–7 March 1959* (held at Walter Reed Army Institute of Research). Washington, DC: U.S. Government Printing Office.

White, M. (1970). Psychological and social barriers to women in science. *Science, 170,* 413–416.

Name Index

Subject Index

DATE DUE

RE	JAN 23 1995	1995	